BLUE MIND, BOLD HEART

ONE MAN. ONE BOAT. ONE LIFE-CHANGING LOOP.

MICHAEL TACKETT

Book Design by Hmdpublishing

CONTENTS

PROLOGUE: THE SPARK

First Light

On April 8, 2024, I sat on the aft deck of our boat, somewhere in Georgia, and watched the sun rise over the water.

Two months into our Great Loop adventure, these early hours had become my quiet ritual—uncharted moments before the world woke up.

It was divinely silent. Just the gentle rhythm of ripples against the hull and a horizon slowly catching fire.

Sunsets are dramatic, but mornings—mornings are sacred.

There's a kind of magic in the stillness, a hush that feels older than time. Birds stirred in the marsh grass. Fish broke the surface like small epiphanies. The light didn't rush; it revealed.

And in that slow unveiling, I felt it: the holy weight of a beginning. The quiet genesis of a new day. Not just the start of another morning—but of something deeper. Something awakening in me.

That morning in Georgia felt like the middle of something profound. But to understand why it mattered, we need to go back to where it began.

Three Months Earlier

On February 3, 2024, my wife, Joanne, and I bought a 40-foot boat and set out on the trip of a lifetime. It didn't disappoint.

It didn't begin with a grand sendoff or a TV-worthy moment of triumph. There was no champagne smashed against the hull, no drone footage of us slipping into the horizon.

Just the two of us—nervous, a little giddy—casting off from a dock in Destin, Florida, into the unknown. We had no idea what we were getting ourselves into. And that was kind of the point.

For 40 years, I'd run the rat race—doing what was expected, building a business, ticking boxes.

I wasn't unhappy, exactly. But somewhere along the way, I had gone numb.

Life had flattened into a loop of its own: emails, errands, meetings, bills, repeat. I was existing. Maintaining. And I could feel something inside me slipping into sleep.

When the Soul Stirs

There come moments in life when transition is no longer a choice—it's a quiet inevitability. For some, it arrives with a jolt: a job loss, a cross-country move, or the kids leaving home.

But for me, it wasn't triggered by a single seismic event. It was more subtle, more internal. A slow erosion of joy.

A deep-seated realization that my sense of yearning—for purpose, for vitality, for life itself—was starting to fade.

Nothing was obviously wrong. From the outside, my life looked perfectly fine. But inside, something essential was quietly slipping away—and I could no longer pretend not to notice.

I've always been a dreamer. A risk-taker. But I had reached a point where nothing was nourishing the deepest parts of me. Life was beginning to feel dangerously shallow.

I'm not talking about my connection to God in a purely spiritual sense. I was searching for something more layered—a triangular relationship between God, His creation, and my own spirit.

My personality has always craved depth. I've never been satisfied with surface-level impressions; I long to experience things fully, to feel them in my bones, to understand them with empathy and wonder.

While my spiritual life was steady, what I lacked was a sense of wholeness—a full comprehension of life itself.

For me, a "full life" meant integration. Call it "3-D" living if you like.

It meant aligning my relationship with God (spirit) and my experience of the world He created (creation) in a way that gave rise to something deeper: a whole, fully alive, and integrated soul.

I believe the soul is formed in the space where our spirit meets and wrestles with the physical world. It's the bridge between heaven and earth—and I was longing to strengthen it.

I needed a jolt. A spark. Something bold enough to wake me up.

What I needed wasn't just a change of scenery. I needed a renewal of the soul.

And that's exactly what I found.

The Quiet Seed

I first discovered America's Great Loop about fifteen years earlier. I was browsing in a bookstore—back when people still did that—and a title caught my eye: *Honey, Let's Get a Boat: A Cruising Adventure of America's Great Loop* by Ron and Eva Stob.

As I read, I was drawn into a 6,000-mile waterway that traces a looping path around the eastern half of North America.

Since the day I first read that book, I was enamored. Something about the adventure lodged in my heart and stayed there. I kept thinking about it. Kept talking about it. Sometimes out loud. Sometimes just to myself.

With no firsthand experience, I had only my imagination to picture what locks, canals, and tidal changes might really be like.

I fantasized about the winding rivers, the quiet anchorages, the freedom of moving with the weather instead of the clock. I wasn't sure I'd ever actually do it, but the dream kept tugging at me.

(What is "The Loop"? Check out: www.youtube.com/watch?v=97YH18DC9mQ)

Years passed. Life got busy. I chased other goals, ran businesses, raised a family. But the Loop never really left me.

Eventually, dreaming wasn't enough. I started planning—and then, I started talking.

Telling people about this 6,000-mile waterway loop that circumnavigates the eastern U.S.—up the Intracoastal Waterway, through the Great Lakes, down the inland rivers, and across the Gulf.

Most people nodded politely, the way you do when someone shares a dream you assume they'll never chase.

I don't blame them. We all carry those kinds of dreams—half-whispered longings we rarely speak aloud. But this one wouldn't go away.

It kept surfacing—on quiet evenings, during long drives, in moments when I asked myself if this was really all there was.

From Dream to Decision

The dream started feeling real the day I stumbled onto YouTube channels like *Sailing Zatara* and *Scho and Jo.*

Sailing Zatara came first—Keith and Renee, a bold and inspiring couple sailing the world with their kids. Their journey wasn't the Loop, but it resonated deeply with me. They had traded normal life for ocean horizons and raw adventure.

As I watched their weekly episodes, I could barely sit still. I longed for the kind of release they had so boldly claimed.

Their voyages became a ritual in our home. Joanne and I would watch over dinner or curled up on the couch, imagining what it might feel like to untie the lines and chase the horizon.

Then we discovered *Scho and Jo,* a couple tackling the Great Loop with zero boating experience. No maritime pedigree, no captain's license—just a dream and a camera. And that made it even more compelling.

Because suddenly, this wasn't just entertainment. It was a blueprint. We saw ourselves in them—not because we knew what we were doing, but because we didn't.

That was the point.

They gave us permission to believe the dream didn't have to stay theoretical. That it was possible to learn as you go—to grow into a new life, even if you weren't born into it.

Eventually, the question stopped being "Could we?" and became "Why not?"

More Than a Vacation

I'll admit, at first, I imagined the Loop as a kind of extended vacation. A slow-motion sightseeing tour. Sunsets at anchor. Drinks on the flybridge. And yes, there was plenty of that.

But there was also docking in crosswinds, engine trouble at inopportune times, emotional fatigue, and moments when I wondered what on earth we'd gotten ourselves into.

The Loop, I came to realize, is not a cruise. It's a crucible. It burns away assumptions. It reveals truths. It demands presence. And in return, it gives you something that few modern experiences offer: clarity.

Clarity about what matters. Clarity about who you are. Clarity about what you're carrying—and what you need to lay down.

The Loop as Mirror

The Great Loop has a way of revealing things. The water doesn't lie. It reflects you. Sometimes gently, sometimes uncomfortably.

It showed me the patterns I'd built to cope with stress. It surfaced the places where my marriage needed stronger lines and better communication. It reminded me, again and again, that I wasn't in control—and that was okay.

Before we even crossed our wake, I realized this wasn't just a trip. It was a mirror. A classroom. A calling.

Each mile chipped away at the version of me I thought I had to be. And in that space, something softer, stronger, and more grounded began to emerge.

Why This Book Exists

This book isn't a cruising guide. It's not a list of marinas or restaurants. It's a field guide for the soul—for anyone who's ever stood at the edge of a bold decision and wondered if they had the courage to jump.

Blue Mind, Bold Heart is about that jump. About the fears that precede it. The faith that fuels it. And the freedom that follows.

This book doesn't follow our route mile by mile. The Great Loop unfolded in a straight line on the water, but my transformation did not. Growth tends to circle back on itself — just like the Loop. So the story drifts through time, revisiting places and people as the lessons reveal themselves.

It's about more than just the miles. It's about changing your interior map. Your sense of direction. Your definition of *home*.

This book is my attempt to capture that shift.

It's about finding stillness in motion, wonder in the ordinary, and transformation in tide and time.

The Invitation

I didn't set out to find myself on America's Great Loop. I just wanted to take an exciting voyage. But somewhere between the docks and the dolphins, the diesel fumes and the quiet mornings on glassy water, I realized I wasn't just cruising. Something else was surfacing.

It wasn't something I could see at the start—and maybe you won't either. But if you take this journey with me, I think you'll begin to feel it too.

The real meaning of this trip didn't reveal itself until the end—and once it did, I couldn't ignore it.

As you read, I think you'll feel it rising—subtle at first, like a ripple building into a wave.

By the time we cross our wake, I hope it lands with you the way it finally did with me. Because once you see it... you can't unsee it. And it might just change the way you chase whatever comes next.

So, whether you're dreaming of your own Loop, wondering what's next, or simply hungry for a deeper current in your life—welcome aboard.

This story is for you.

LOOP LESSONS – THE SPARK

Stillness is sacred. The quiet of early mornings on the water has the power to stir something eternal within us. Listen to what rises in the silence.

Numbness is a warning sign. When life becomes a loop of maintenance instead of meaning, it's time to wake up and reevaluate.

True change begins within. Not all turning points come with fanfare. Some arrive in whispers—a slow erosion of joy that signals it's time for something deeper.

Spiritual wholeness requires integration. The soul forms when spirit and creation collide—when your inner life and outer experience align in wonder and presence.

Dreams grow quietly. A single book or video can plant a seed. What seems like a passing curiosity may turn out to be your next calling.

You don't need credentials to begin. You don't have to be a seasoned mariner to chase the Loop—or any big dream. Willingness matters more than expertise.

The Loop is more than a route. It's a crucible that refines identity, peels back pretense, and gives clarity about what really matters.

Life is spiritual, even when it's physical. The boat, the water, the sunrise—these aren't just logistics. They're language. Pay attention to what they're saying.

Start before you're ready. There will never be a perfect moment to leap. But there *is* a moment when the ache to stay stuck becomes louder than the fear to move forward. That's when it's time.

Follow the spark. When something lights up your soul, trust it. Even if it scares you. Especially if it scares you.

CHAPTER 01
WHAT'S JIMMY BUFFETT GOT TO DO WITH IT?

September 2, 2023 Like most mornings, I woke early, checked my email, and scrolled through the news. That's when I saw it: Jimmy Buffett had died late the night before.

It hit hard—shocking, but not entirely unexpected. The man who'd spent a lifetime chasing the sun had finally run out of daylight.

I went to the lake alone that morning and stared out over the water. It felt stiller than usual, like even the breeze was holding its breath.

I couldn't help but wonder: *When will my appointment with death come?* And more importantly, *how will I spend the time between now and then?*

That morning on the lake, something inside me cracked. Buffett's death wasn't just a headline—it was a mirror.

While he'd lived wide open, I had recently begun to shrink my world, grinding myself down for reasons I couldn't even name anymore.

I had already hit my limit. For months, I couldn't shake a line from Buffett's *Trying to Reason with Hurricane Season* that said he couldn't keep up his pace much longer. It was the quiet anthem of my unraveling.

I was exhausted—physically, mentally, spiritually—and running on fumes with no refuel in sight. His death didn't cause my burnout, but it spotlighted it, made it impossible to ignore.

The truth was painful: I was slowly killing myself with stress, all while willingly settling into a life of comfort.

But deep down, I knew I needed something radically different. That was the moment I had to choose.

I had always marched to my own beat, but even with my adventurous and unpredictable personality, I had fallen into familiar and comfortable patterns. I had played my part well, checking the boxes, meeting the deadlines, building the life that looked good from the outside.

But now, inside, something was unsettled. A quiet ache. A sense that I had stepped away from my roots of living true to myself. Standing there, staring at the horizon—or maybe just at the stretch of water ahead—I could feel the weight of that choice.

One path led deeper into the familiar, into the well-worn grooves of a life now settling into comfort and ease.

The other was uncertain, uncharted, and a little terrifying. But it was mine. That part felt exhilarating, more like the 'me' I loved.

To write my own story would mean letting go of some things. Control. The illusion of certainty. Traditional living. It would mean stepping into discomfort, into mistakes, into growth. It would mean listening to the voice that had been recently whispering: *There's more.*

That was the moment I knew: It was time to break out of the 'normal' and get back to living on my own terms.

The Adventure

The Loop wasn't just a boating trip—it became a lifeline. A way to reclaim wonder, breathe again, and rediscover who I was outside the grind.

It offered something the normal world couldn't: space to be still, to move with purpose, and to live by the rhythm of tides instead of calendars. So, I stopped hesitating.

The dream that had waited patiently in the background became a plan. My excitement for the Great Loop—the one that had been simmering for years—started to roar.

Five months later, almost to the day, we bought the boat. Three days after that, we left the dock, the dream became reality.

Every Looper has a story—a moment, a spark, a turning point that set them on this path. There's always something that nudges them out of the ordinary and into the extraordinary.

I'm not talking about the lifelong mariners who've always lived near water and made boating second nature. I mean the rest of us—those who didn't grow up in marinas or charting courses, but who felt something shift.

For most Loopers, something either clicked... or something broke. For me, it was both. Something clicked—and something broke.

The click was the realization that life was passing me by while I checked boxes that no longer meant anything. The break was quieter, more personal: a slow unraveling of identity, purpose, and energy.

I wasn't depressed exactly—but I was depleted. Worn thin by expectations I no longer believed in, chasing goals that no longer inspired me.

The Loop didn't feel like a vacation. It felt like an escape route. Not from responsibility, but from a version of myself I couldn't carry anymore.

And in that breaking, something beautiful began—the kind of freedom that can only come when you're finally willing to let go.

Unplugging from Dirt Life

I first heard the term "dirt life" while docked at Jekyll Island, Georgia. That's where we met Mark and Terry—and their dog, Annie—aboard *Annie Marie*.

They were the first real Looper friends we made, and though we didn't travel together the entire way, we ended up sharing 395 miles of water and friendship.

One evening during docktails, Mark casually mentioned how strange it was to be away from "dirt life"—his way of describing life on land. The phrase struck me immediately. It captured something essential.

Life on land is often seen as secure, predictable, grounded—"keep your feet on the ground," as the old saying goes. But water life is the opposite: fluid, uncertain, thrilling. It invites you to drift, explore, and let go.

Mark was one Looper who is the perfect picture of joy. I didn't know Mark prior to the Loop, so I can't say if the Loop changed him or not, but man, what a happy guy! He and Terry crossed their wake in May 2025.

I spoke to him recently and he, like me, is struggling with returning to the dirt--some of us just can't wrap our heads around going back, or as it seems, "backwards".

There's something about the water that gets in your soul and doesn't let go.

I never realized just how "dirty" land-life could be—not in the literal sense, but in how cluttered and tangled it becomes. We get caught up in activities, obligations, relationships, and routines that don't always serve our well-being.

Preparing for the Loop forced me to take a hard look at all of it.

Unplugging from dirt life was far more difficult than I imagined. We had to unravel layers of commitments—church, clubs, volunteer work, family duties. Every bill had to be canceled or moved to autopay. The cars needed a plan. We needed someone we trusted to handle local issues while we were gone.

What I thought would be a simple transition turned out to be a full-on unwinding of a life too busy to breathe.

For other reasons, we had sold our home the previous August, which made the idea of taking on the Loop more viable. But we hadn't fully committed.

That changed when Buffett passed. His death was the spark that lit the fuse.

It wasn't a sudden impulse—but in that moment, the balance finally tipped. The excuses faded. The dream that had long been simmering beneath the surface surged to the top, and I knew: it was time.

As we disconnected from one life to step into another, it hit me just how entangling modern living had become. No wonder so few people actually do this trip. The logistics alone are enough to scare you back into routine.

Fewer people complete the Great Loop each year than summit Mount Everest—a fact that still surprises me. While Everest sees around 800 successful summits annually, fewer than 250 boats typically complete the Loop each year.

In 2022, 227 boats crossed their wake, setting a record at the time. That record was broken again in 2024, (our fleet) with 270 completions—still a small number in the grand scheme of things.

Despite being far less publicized than Everest, the Loop remains a rare and demanding journey. It may not involve high altitudes or ice axes—none of which I have any desire to take on—but the Loop demands a different kind of endurance: mental, emotional, and relational.

And anyone who's completed it will tell you the same thing—it transforms you just as profoundly.

The Reactions

When we told people about our plans, the responses ran the gamut. Most smiled politely, but I could tell they thought we were crazy.

Some clearly doubted we'd even go through with it, their expressions betraying more than their words. A few voiced concerns that the journey would prove too hard or that we'd be disappointed. Others thought it was an exciting adventure—but only for someone else.

More than a few warned it might be too dangerous, citing everything from unpredictable weather to mechanical breakdowns.

And then, thankfully, there were the believers. Those rare souls who simply said, "Go for it." They saw the dream for what it was and encouraged us to chase it.

Starting the Loop means swimming through a sea of doubters, skeptics, and well-meaning voices that echo their own fear back at you. You have to keep your course anyway.

Let me offer you some encouragement as you face the doubters: if you choose to take on the Loop, you'll quickly discover you're not alone. All along the route, you'll find others who made the same hard choices, carried the weight of preparation, and pushed past doubt to chase something more.

And their stories—ordinary people doing extraordinary things—are nothing short of inspiring.

In South Carolina at the Swansboro Town Docks, we met Karl on *Callie B*, a man who completed the Loop solo on his Sea Ray 400. I still don't know how he navigated over 100 locks single-handed.

And then there was the couple in their mid-90s we met in Orange Beach, just as we were wrapping up our own Loop—living proof that age doesn't have to anchor your dreams.

Stories like theirs are everywhere out here, quiet reminders that the human spirit still burns bright in those who choose to live fully. I was proud to be counted among them.

Their courage, kindness, and camaraderie became a lifeline—holding me up, holding me in—as we became part of this remarkable floating community.

The truth is, you don't find yourself on the Loop because you're chasing photo ops. You're here because you refuse to settle. As Jimmy

Buffett once sang, he'd rather fully live than drift through life half-dead. That's the heart of it. That's the call I answered.

Get Busy Living

What started as a daring adventure quickly became a master class in personal growth. The first and most important lesson was simple but urgent: just do it.

Life isn't meant to be spent merely surviving—it's meant to be lived fully, without waiting for the 'right time' that never comes.

What taking the plunge and doing the Loop taught us was that we had grown complacent with living. We weren't learning new things anymore. The routine of daily life had dulled our sense of wonder.

But once we cast off, we rediscovered that experiencing the unknown is the true essence of living. It awakened a spirit of discovery inside us that we hadn't felt in years.

If there's a single message the Loop etched into us, it's this: get busy living or accept that you are already dead.

We also discovered how cluttered our lives had become. As we unplugged, it became clear how many obligations, tasks, and distractions drained our time and energy without returning any joy or purpose.

It was a wake-up call to simplify and refocus. Along the way, we learned to tune out the voices of doubt—especially from those who didn't share our vision. Their reasons for hesitation were often just fear disguised as wisdom.

Another revelation came from an old Buffett lyric, about regretting it if you ended up living a lie. The trip exposed some uncomfortable truths about how I had been living—truths I could finally face with honesty and grace.

And finally, preparing to leave showed me how many invisible lines were tethering me to the dock. Cutting those lines wasn't easy, but it was liberating in the deepest sense. Each step toward departure became a cleansing of the soul, a shedding of what no longer served us.

No matter who you are, you become numb to life if you don't constantly introduce new experiences. The Loop made this crystal clear.

Jimmy Buffett never knew me—but the way he lived stirred something in me. His life gave me the courage to dream differently, and his death reminded me that time doesn't wait.

The day he died, I stopped waiting and got back to living.

I hope he'd be pleased. I know I am.

The rest of this book will share what the journey taught me—the lessons learned from 6,000 miles on the water, and the deeper currents beneath the surface.

LESSONS LEARNED FROM "WHAT'S JIMMY BUFFETT GOT TO DO WITH IT?"

Mortality is a mirror. The news of a hero's death can force you to examine how you're spending your own limited time.

Burnout is a warning light, not a badge of honor. Exhaustion—physical, mental, spiritual—signals that something fundamental must change.

You can trade society's script for your own story. Life isn't about meeting external expectations; it's about writing a narrative that feels authentic.

Adventure can be a lifeline. The Loop offered space to breathe, wonder, and live by tides rather than calendars.

Big decisions often start with a single spark. Buffett's passing turned a long-held dream into an urgent plan.

"Dirt life" is comfortable but numbing. Routine on land can dull curiosity; water life reawakens it.

Unplugging is harder than it looks—but worth the hassle. Canceling obligations, automating bills, and selling a house are heavy lifts that create room for freedom.

Logistics deter most dreamers. The complexity of leaving "normal life" explains why so few people ever cast off.

Expect skepticism—and sail anyway. Doubters, worriers, and armchair critics will appear; their fears reflect their limits, not yours.

Surround yourself with believers. Encouragement from even a few "Go for it!" voices can drown out a sea of doubt.

"Just do it" beats "someday." Waiting for the perfect moment keeps dreams on hold indefinitely.

Novelty is nourishment. Regular doses of the unknown keep the mind sharp and the spirit alive.

Clutter—physical and mental—quietly steals joy. Shedding tasks, stuff, and distractions reveals what truly matters.

Doubt often disguises itself as wisdom. People's warnings are frequently fear in respectable clothing.

Authenticity prevents regret. Living a lie eventually catches up with you; better to face hard truths now.

Invisible lines can hold you to the dock. Until you cut ties that no longer serve you, real departure is impossible.

Role models matter—even from afar. Buffett never knew you, but his example showed that bold, joyful living is possible.

New experiences keep you alive; complacency equals slow death. You're either busy discovering—or busy eroding.

The decision to leave was just the beginning. What followed was a journey that tested, stretched, and ultimately transformed us. In the next chapter, we take the plunge—literally.

CHAPTER 02
THE DREAM THAT TOOK SHAPE

June 10, 2024

We were four months into the Loop, pushing north along the Atlantic coast. Our destination that day: Manasquan, New Jersey.

Joanne and I had left Atlantic City aboard *PATIENCE,* our 40-foot cruiser, under a forecast that promised "moderate seas." But by now, I'd learned the hard truth of marine weather: forecasts are polite suggestions, not promises.

And that morning, the sea had something else in mind.

Spray flew over the bow in sheets as *PATIENCE* slammed into the chop, bucking and twisting like a rodeo bronc.

Every jolt rattled the hull and my nerves. The wheel strained in my hands as I tried to hold course. I was tense but focused—until I heard Joanne's voice cut through the wind from the back deck:

"The dinghy's in the water!"

My gut dropped.

We kept a small inflatable tender strapped to the swim platform—our ride to shore when we anchored out. It was always secured with a system of tie-down straps and steel brackets.

I snapped the helm into autopilot and raced aft.

Sure enough, the brackets had bent under pressure, and two of the straps had failed. Our dinghy was no longer riding snug against the stern. It was half-submerged, thrashing wildly in the water—still tethered, but just barely.

The outboard motor was getting mercilessly dunked with every passing swell, slamming sideways into the back of the boat. The whole thing looked like it might tear off and vanish into the sea at any moment.

"Turn us to port!" I yelled to Joanne. "Try to turn us—get the seas following instead of hitting us on the beam!

As she jumped to the helm, I dropped to my knees and crawled onto the slick swim platform—waves washing over it, threatening to knock me clean off.

Salt spray stung my eyes. The deck pitched beneath me like a seesaw.

I clung to the rail, then reached out to wrestle the dinghy's motor upright—desperate to at least minimize the damage.

But each time I got it near vertical, a wave would crash and knock it back again, drenching me and slamming the engine deeper into the water.

I finally threw a fresh strap over the dinghy's frame and cinched it as tight as I could, locking it down to ride out the waves. But I knew the truth: the motor was already waterlogged, maybe ruined.

Our buddy boat, *Soul of a Sailor*, was trailing about 300 yards behind. Through binoculars, they watched the entire mess unfold in real time. From their perspective, it must've looked like a man hanging off the stern of a pitching boat, dangerously close to disaster.

And honestly? That's exactly what it was.

There was nothing more to do. Soaked, frustrated, and humbled, I climbed back to the helm and did the only thing left: I kept us pointed north.

For three more hours, I watched that poor dinghy get dragged through a minefield of waves—twisting, slamming, threatening to shear off with each swell.

By the time we reached Manasquan and tied up, I was wrecked.

Soul of a Sailor docked beside us. Chad, the captain—and by then, a trusted friend—walked over to survey the damage. We stood together at the stern, looking down at the battered tender and the mangled engine.

He shook his head. "That could've ended a lot worse," he said. "I'll help you get it secured... but that engine's toast."

Then he looked me straight in the eye. His voice shifted, lower now. "You know what really concerns me?"

I waited.

"You were on that swim platform. In those seas. And you weren't wearing a PFD" (personal flotation device).

I ran the scene back in my mind. He was right. I hadn't. My heart sank.

"Oh my gosh," I said quietly. "I didn't."

He didn't lecture. He didn't need to. The look in his eyes said everything. That kind of mistake doesn't need a second chance.

"That won't happen again," I said. And I meant it.

So how does a 62-year-old man end up off the coast of New Jersey, wrestling a half-drowned dinghy on a rolling deck?

It all started with one seemingly random decision: picking up that little book with the quirky title—*Honey, Let's Get a Boat*. Funny how a single moment like that can quietly alter the course of your life.

That dream—conceived in a bookstore and fanned into flame by YouTube and quiet longing—had finally taken shape.

Before I take you into the heart of our journey, there's one question I get asked more than any other: *"What exactly is the Great Loop?"*

The Route

For the sake of clarity—especially if you've never heard of the Great Loop—here's how it works:

Most Loopers start somewhere in Florida or on the East Coast and travel **counterclockwise** to take advantage of the river currents. The journey follows:

The Atlantic Intracoastal Waterway (ICW) north from Florida to New York

The Hudson River, then either the **Erie Canal** or the **Champlain route** into Canada

The Trent-Severn Waterway across Ontario to the Georgian Bay and North Channel

The Great Lakes, mostly Lake Michigan

The Inland Rivers (Illinois, Mississippi, Ohio, Cumberland, and Tennessee)

The Gulf of Mexico and back along the **Gulf Intracoastal Waterway** to Florida

You can take detours. You can linger. You can loop in pieces or all at once. There's no one right way to do it. That's part of the beauty.

Loopers identify each other by the **burgee**—a white triangular flag that means "currently looping."

Once you finish and cross your wake—return to where you started—you earn the **gold burgee**. It's a small piece of fabric, but it carries the weight of thousands of miles, lessons, storms, and memories.

The America's Great Loop Cruisers Association (AGLCA) is the unofficial hub of this community. They provide resources, host events, and connect boaters who are somewhere along the route—or dreaming about it.

But charts and guidebooks can only tell you so much. They don't cover what happens in the miles between the marinas. They don't tell you how it will undo you in some places... and remake you in others.

It will test your marriage, your patience, your confidence, and your boat. And somewhere along the way, you'll realize: this was never just about boating. You'll navigate through fog, locks, currents, and conversations with fellow cruisers from all walks of life.

And if you let it, the Loop will change you.

It will cast aside baggage you didn't know you were carrying. It will quiet the noise of a land-bound life and hand you back the sound of your own thoughts.

The rhythm of the water will replace the rhythm of the clock. Your days will center around weather, tides, fuel, food, and anchorage—not emails and meetings.

It's not just a voyage around America. It's a voyage into yourself.

If you've ever longed to trade the noise for something quieter, simpler, deeper—then maybe it's time to follow your own version of the Loop.

LOOP LESSONS: THE DREAM THAT TOOK SHAPE

Loop Lessons: The Dream That Took Shape

Always wear a PFD—especially in rough seas. Safety is never optional.

Forecasts are suggestions. The ocean decides.

Boating humbles you. Often with saltwater. Sometimes with silence.

Big dreams often begin in quiet places—a book, a video, a passing thought.

The Loop is not about perfection. It's about persistence, presence, and learning.

You'll fix things you've never fixed before—on the boat and in yourself.

You'll be tested: your marriage, your patience, your confidence, your systems.

What feels like a crisis may become your most memorable classroom.

The journey may circle a continent—but it also leads inward.

It's never just about boating. It's about becoming.

CHAPTER 03
THE RHYTHM OF PATIENCE

If I had to point to one simple thing that captures just how deeply the Loop affected me, it's this: it changed the way I experience time.

The Loop taught me to measure life in miles, not minutes—in seasons, not days. Covering 40 miles on the water takes a full day; by car, it would take less than an hour. Out here, you can't live by the same clock that governs life on land. Weather, tides, and currents set the rhythm. Plans become suggestions. Flexibility becomes a survival skill.

And maybe most of all, the Loop begins to teach you something that modern life rarely does: the value of waiting. Not just waiting, but waiting well.

For me, the real impact—the heart of the Loop Effect—was realizing that time itself shifts on the water. It stretches. It softens. It demands patience.

And in that quiet space between rushing and resting, it makes room for what truly matters.

How PATIENCE Got Her Name

You might think naming our boat would've been the easy part. After all, I'd spent nearly 15 years dreaming about the Loop, planning each detail in my mind—but I could never settle on a name. Somehow, that decision kept eluding me.

It wasn't until we actually bought her that the name finally came.

We were sitting at McGuire's Irish Pub in Destin, Florida, celebrating the purchase, when the word just slipped out. "Patience," I said aloud, almost to myself.

Joanne looked up. "You definitely need patience—but what are you talking about?"

She wasn't wrong. Patience and I had never been well acquainted.

Over the course of our marriage, Joanne had gently—and sometimes not so gently—reminded me that waiting, resting, and surrendering control didn't come naturally to me. Even preparing for the Loop had tested every ounce of patience I had.

But that night, the name settled over me like truth. "Patience," I repeated. "That's it. That's her name." It wasn't just a label—it was a lesson. A mantra. A daily reminder of what I was trying to become.

Every time I called her name over the radio, every time I introduced her in a marina, I'd be reminding myself of the deeper reason I was out here.

Joanne nodded, and with that, the boat had her name—and I had a quiet compass by which to steer.

LAND LIFE

I started working young and figured out pretty quickly that I wasn't built for a time clock. My first job was on a ranch in California at sixteen.

After we moved to Tennessee, I graduated early and started college just before my seventeenth birthday.

From that point on, I chased independence. I launched my first business during college and never really stopped.

Over the years, Joanne and I ran everything from investment-related firms to rental properties to renewable energy ventures—always preferring the freedom (and chaos) of self-employment.

I tried traditional employment once—took an advertising job at a local newspaper. I was good at it, but the obsession with hours and structure drove me crazy. I lasted exactly 30 days before tossing my keys on the desk and walking out.

That brief brush with corporate life only confirmed what I already knew: I was meant to chart my own course. And maybe that's part of what drew me to the Loop.

Out there, like in business, you sink or swim based on your own decisions—and no one's watching the clock.

TIME AND PERFORMANCE

I think that's part of what drew me to the water—and to the Loop. Life out there runs on a different paradigm. Time takes a back seat to performance. You can't rush on the water without risking real consequences.

Some of the biggest trouble people encounter on the Loop can be traced back to one thing: a schedule.

That's why, when planning to meet up with guests, seasoned Loopers will say, "I can give you a place or a time—but not both."

Trying to force the trip into a calendar box leads to bad decisions. You push through when you should wait. You head out in rough seas, or you try to dock when the wind and current say otherwise. And sometimes, the cost isn't just a dented ego or scratched gelcoat.

Sometimes, it's your life.

More than once, we were delayed for days—whether in Fort Pierce waiting on weather, or on the Erie Canal riding out a hurricane's remnants. Out here, patience isn't optional—it's a way of life.

Out here, you can't live by the calendar the way you do on land. You're directed by things beyond your control. You move according to circumstances, not schedules. You learn to respond rather than resist. You get in rhythm with the moment instead of fighting it.

There's a funny saying among Loopers—when someone asks what day it is, the answer is often, "It's *Blursday.*"

It's not just a joke; it's a blessing. It means you've finally slipped free of the tyranny of the calendar.

It reminds me of a Kenny Chesney lyric about not really knowing what day it is after rocking for many days in a row.

I get it, Kenny. I really do. That kind of blurry, timeless rhythm becomes normal out here.

But I'll be honest—slipping into that rhythm didn't come naturally to me. I've always admired people who could bend circumstances to their will.

That used to be my default setting. You can get away with that on the Loop for a little while... but eventually, it catches up with you.

And that's not just a cruising truth—it's a life truth. The strongest people aren't the ones who power through everything; they're the ones who know when to wait, when to yield, and when to move with the current instead of against it.

Stop measuring life by minutes and hours. Start experiencing it through seasons, milestones, and joy. After all, there's a reason the word "deadline" begins with *"dead."*

"PATIENCE" It wasn't just the name of our boat—it was the lesson I kept learning, wave after wave.

One last thought—something Jimmy Buffett wrote has stuck with me for years. Everyone knows *Come Monday,* the love song he penned for his wife, Jane, early in their marriage.

But it's the follow-up song, *"Coast of Carolina,"* written much later, that really hits home for me. In it, he reflects on the trials and triumphs of a long relationship. There's a line in that song that stops me every time, about walls that you can't seem to ever break down.

Some walls in life aren't meant to be knocked down. Some problems just won't budge. You can either keep bruising yourself trying to tear them down—or you can choose a different approach.

You can learn to live with them, dress them up with grace, humor, or even gratitude. Or you can climb—use them to rise.

These days, my life feels lighter because I've stopped swinging the hammer. I've learned to accept what can't be changed, to see the value in what once frustrated me.

Some of those walls have even become familiar—almost welcome. They remind me I'm human. And that sometimes, peace doesn't come from solving the problem, but from changing how you live with it.

Learning to live with life's limits didn't mean giving up—it meant shifting gears. And once I embraced that truth, I knew it was time to act.

TIME TO ACT — Before the Clock Runs Out

Kenny Chesney nails a universal truth in one line in "*Beer in Mexico*" where he reminds us that time goes by fast. Blink, and decades disappear.

I felt that sting when I realized 62 birthdays had slipped past like mile-markers on the Intracoastal Waterway. It's why I told Joanne, "We're not getting younger. If we don't cast off now, we may never do it."

So, we did the Loop—because waiting another season wasn't an option.

Now I'm asking you: *What dream keeps tugging at your sleeve?* What adventure, business, song, or book have you shelved for "someday"? The calendar is relentless, and every tick narrows your choices.

Stop negotiating with the clock. Trade hesitation for motion, plans for wake, and fear for the thrill of open water—whatever "open water" looks like in your life. Because the minutes will pass, no matter what—so let them pass with salt spray on your face, purpose in your heart, and the quiet strength of *patience* guiding you forward, one meaningful mile at a time.

LOOP LESSONS – THE RHYTHM OF PATIENCE

The water runs on its own time. Out here, you don't control the pace—weather, tides, and currents do. You learn to adjust, not resist.

Patience is a practice, not a personality trait. You're not born with it—you build it, one delay and detour at a time.

Life moves in seasons, not seconds. Boating forces you to slow down, stretch time, and live in rhythm instead of on schedule.

Waiting well is its own kind of motion. Sometimes progress isn't about speed—it's about alignment, wisdom, and timing.

Forcing a schedule often leads to regret. The most common Looping mistakes happen when we push instead of pause.

Let go of the land-clock. Out here, days blur and deadlines vanish. That's not laziness—it's liberation.

True power is knowing when not to act. Yielding to the moment, riding the wave, and choosing peace over push is strength, not weakness.

PATIENCE isn't just a name—it's a navigational tool. When the world demands you rush, patience becomes the quiet compass that keeps you safe, steady, and sane.

Time is not your enemy—it's your teacher. It reveals your priorities, reshapes your pace, and reminds you what's worth the wait.

CHAPTER 04
UNCHARTED WATERS

Departure

February 6, 2024—that was the day it all began. We pulled away from Destin, Florida, officially launching our Great Loop adventure.

It wasn't the champagne-and-confetti sendoff I'd imagined. Instead, we fumbled out of the slip, tension thick in the air, as if even the boat could sense our inexperience.

The strain between Joanne and me surfaced almost immediately, setting the tone for a journey that would test us far beyond navigation and miles.

For better or for worse, we were officially "on the Loop".

As we made our way from Destin, Florida to Panama City, along the Intracoastal Waterway (ICW), my mind kept drifting back to the day months earlier when I sat by the lake pondering my future.

That day, I'd made an impulsive decision to commit to this trip—diving headfirst into something I barely understood. Joanne, on the other hand, had been nervous from the start.

That moment revealed just how differently we approached life: me, the risk-taker chasing a dream, and her, the realist weighing the consequences, but fully supportive. This trip was going to expose those differences in powerful ways, and help us to understand each other at a new depth.

In those first few days, everything felt unfamiliar—how the boat handled, how to read the water, even how we communicated under pressure. We were stepping into entirely new roles, and the learning curve was steep.

The stress showed up in small ways at first: missed cues, tense silences, a sharp word here or there.

But beneath it all, we were both committed to figuring it out. We just didn't yet know how much the Loop would ask of us—or teach us.

Seventy-three miles later, we pulled into Emerald Harbor Marina in Panama City. It's hard to put into words what it feels like to approach your very first dock completely on your own. Joanne had called ahead and reserved us a spot, but I didn't learn our slip assignment until we were just five minutes out.

I hailed the marina and was told we'd be on a T-head. "Thank God," I thought, breathing a little easier. At least I wouldn't have to squeeze this big girl into a narrow slip on day one.

Another unexpected blessing came in the form of a fellow Looper who came running down to catch our lines. I'm embarrassed to say I never got his name, but in that moment, he was a lifeline.

His simple act of kindness confirmed what we had hoped: the Looper family was real—and they'd be there when we needed them.

I'm the kind of person who learns best by doing. Traditional classroom learning never really worked for me—I lasted about two years in college before boredom set in, and I wasn't any wiser for the effort.

So, when it came time to chase the Loop, I took the same approach: jump in, figure it out along the way.

Seasoned boaters—and wise ones, I'll admit—often warn against simply casting off and learning as you go. But that's exactly what we did. I had never docked a 40-foot boat until three days before we departed.

When I slid her confidently onto that T-head in Panama City, I felt surprisingly capable... and a bit too proud of myself.

The Gulf Crossing

It was the second day in a row we were reminded—uncomfortably—that we were in deep, unfamiliar waters.

Just the day before, we'd anchored off Dog Island—a beautiful, deceptively calm spot that quietly masked the ever-present dangers nearby.

We were staging for the Gulf Crossing, widely considered the most dangerous stretch of the entire Loop: 170 miles of open water, farther offshore than any other leg of the journey.

We were up before dawn, pulling anchor at 5 AM. It was pitch black. I had to rely entirely on my electronics to navigate out of the ICW and into the Gulf.

For seasoned boaters, that might be routine—but for me, it was a first.

The inlet water was choppy, and the darkness only amplified my tension. I inched along at six knots, barely able to see the waves with my bow light.

For two straight hours, I was locked at the helm, eyes glued to the GPS, white-knuckled and praying—truly praying—for daylight.

At first light, I eased her up on plane and settled in around 17 MPH. We ran that way for the next nine hours.

At that point in the journey, we had no Looper friends. No buddy boats. We were crossing solo.

When I later told fellow Loopers about it, I saw it in their eyes: they didn't just think we were foolish—they *knew* we were. And they were right.

The Gulf is not to be underestimated. It can turn fast, and weather forecasts are often optimistic at best.

We made it without incident, but not because of skill or preparation. It was nothing but grace—pure providence—that gave us calm seas and a trouble-free run.

After a few thousand miles and plenty of conversations with seasoned Loopers, I came to see just how reckless that Gulf crossing really was. But in hindsight, it was our baptism by fire.

That day tested both our boat and our nerve—and we made it through.

No matter what the next 5,500 miles would throw at us, we had one solid truth to hold onto: we'd faced the big one early, and we came out the other side.

That counted for something. It still does.

No matter what else can be said about that day, one thing is undeniable: on February 9, 2024, we were fully alive.

Every emotion was raw, every thought focused, every action deliberate. There was no autopilot—only presence, purpose, and the undeniable pulse of being completely in the moment.

Regardless of who you are or how full your life may seem, you start to go numb if you don't continually invite new experiences into your world. The mind dulls, the spirit drifts, and days begin to blend together in a quiet kind of erosion.

The Great Loop made that crystal clear to me.

Every new port, every docking challenge, every unexpected conversation or unfamiliar waterway sparked something awake in me—something I didn't realize had gone quiet back on land.

Adventure, even in small doses, shakes off the rust and reminds you that you're still growing, still changing, still fully alive.

As the shoreline of western Florida came into view, I felt a surge of accomplishment—and a quiet sense of pride. "*Well done,*" I whispered to myself.

I stood a little taller at the helm, riding that wave of confidence as we made our way up the beautiful channel toward the marina.

For a moment, I felt like a seasoned captain.

Tarpon Springs

But that feeling didn't last. We had crossed the Gulf—too early, too alone—and landed in Tarpon Springs, where the unraveling began."

I attempted to dock and delivered what could only be called a controlled crash.

The angle was wrong, the current too strong, and the approach too fast, and it was my confidence that absorbed the brunt of the impact.

Deckhands stood on the T-head, watching with a mix of chuckling and concern as I desperately tried to get PATIENCE to cooperate.

From the bow, Joanne shouted, "You're coming in too hot! Slow down!"

"I've got it!" I snapped back—though clearly, I didn't.

She tried to throw the line to the deckhand, but it caught awkwardly. "You didn't run it under the railing," I growled.

Lines flew, fenders bounced, and I finally got us mostly straight. The deckhands pushed hard against the hull, trying to soften the bump against the pilings.

When the boat was finally tied off and still, silence settled like fog. I looked over at Joanne, expecting her usual calm, but her jaw was tight.

She climbed down from the bow and walked over, voice low. "We need a better plan next time."

"I said I've got it," I muttered, avoiding eye contact.

"No," she replied gently but firmly. "You didn't."

That one stung.

I sighed and leaned against the rail, suddenly tired. "I panicked," I admitted. "Everything I practiced just... vanished."

Joanne's tone softened. "Then let's practice together. You don't have to have it all figured out."

Her words cut through the fog of frustration. She wasn't mad—she was showing up, again, as a partner.

I nodded slowly. "Thanks for not jumping overboard."

She smiled. "Trust me—I thought about it."

We both laughed, and the tension broke.

That evening, I sat quietly on the aft deck, nursing a bruised ego and watching the water shift beneath us.

Doubt crept in, subtle at first, then louder: Had I bitten off more than I could chew? Had I dragged us into something we weren't ready for?

Panic Attack

The next morning took things from shaky to downright terrifying. Around 10 a.m., the dockmaster stopped by to let us know we had to vacate our slip by noon. I wasn't ready—not mentally, not emotionally.

I had hoped for at least a day or two to catch my breath. Instead, I spiraled. Panic set in, unlike anything I'd ever felt. My heart raced, my mind spun. I might've had a full-blown panic attack.

I suddenly doubted everything: Could I even dock on a simple T-head again, let alone navigate into a tight slip?

We had no reservations beyond Tarpon Springs—what if every other marina was full?

Where would we go?

Why hadn't we planned better?

Our inexperience was glaring, and we were utterly alone in it. We'd jumped into the deep end, only to realize we didn't yet know how to swim.

I didn't realize it at the time, but that spiral wasn't the end of something—it was the beginning.

That's how growth works. You face what unnerves you, what scares you sick. And when you come out the other side, you're not the same. You're stronger, wiser—a more complete version of yourself.

The entire trip was to be a journey of firsts—uncharted waters in every sense. We wouldn't spend a single moment retracing our steps.

Each day promised something new: fresh challenges, fresh scenery, new marinas, unknown waterways and constant opportunities to learn and grow.

The Loop takes you through nearly every kind of water imaginable—tidal swings of eleven feet, shallow bays, open Gulf crossings, the vast Great Lakes, and over 100 locks scattered across the Erie Canal and the Trent-Severn Waterway, followed by 1,500 miles down the inland rivers. It was a true test of seamanship.

For us, every day was uncharted territory—and that was exactly the point.

The Loop stripped away the comfort and routine I had grown used to—a life where I could go through the motions half-asleep—and transformed me into someone who had to stay sharp, alert to every detail.

Out here, I was constantly reminded that I didn't even know what I didn't know.

I had pitched the Loop to Joanne as a tour of America—a journey through canals, coasts, and rivers.

But deep down, I'd always known the truth.

It wasn't just about seeing the country.

It was about seeing ourselves.

About gazing into our souls.

LOOP LESSONS FROM UNCHARTED WATERS

New beginnings are rarely picture-perfect. Even long-anticipated adventures can start with stress, doubt, and tension—but that doesn't mean they aren't worthwhile.

Unfamiliar experiences expose hidden insecurities. Inexperience brings vulnerability, and it's easy to misdirect frustration at those closest to you.

Self-awareness is key to healthy relationships. Recognizing when you're projecting your own stress onto others is the first step toward growth.

Small routines can ease big anxieties. Simple habits—like being at the helm 15 minutes before departure—can reduce stress and create harmony.

Even strong marriages can be stretched—and strengthened—by challenge. The Loop required a deeper, more intuitive level of teamwork than anything before.

Trust is built not just over years, but moment by moment. A glance or unspoken understanding between partners becomes essential on the water.

Panic reveals what preparation hides. Stress can surface suddenly—especially when plans fall through—and force you to confront your limitations.

Growth often feels like fear at first. The discomfort of inexperience is what fuels learning and transformation.

Every day on the Loop is a blank slate. The journey offers constant newness: new routes, new water conditions, new lessons.

Adventure shakes off the rust of routine. Without new challenges, life becomes dull—even if it looks full on the outside.

You don't know what you don't know. Humility is essential; you're always learning, and the water has a way of teaching quickly.

The unknown is where growth lives. True transformation requires stepping into unfamiliar territory and learning as you go.

Vulnerability is not weakness—it's a doorway to depth. Letting go of the need to always have it together allows for real connection, both with yourself and others.

Growth comes at the edge of your comfort zone. The Loop doesn't just take you to new places—it stretches who you are. That's the real journey.

CHAPTER 05
LESSONS FROM THE SPILL

They say confession is good for the soul—so let's find out. Just know this before we begin: the engine survived, and so did my ego.

Until now, this story stayed sealed in the bilge where it belonged. But some tales are too messy—and too good—not to share.

It was March 11. We pulled out of the Venetian Marina and Yacht Club, cruising up toward Hollywood Beach to anchor for the night.

My brother Doug and his wife Jana were on board, soaking up the views of million-dollar homes and mega-yachts. Life was good.

Then, at exactly 12:41 p.m.—I have the pictures to prove it—I glanced down at the helm and saw something you never want to see: the port engine oil pressure was reading almost zero.

I handed off the wheel to Doug and bolted below. I swung open the engine room hatch—and froze.

Oil. Everywhere.

The Spill

Back to the bridge. I shut down the **starboard** engine in my panic, then ran back down to double-check.

Wrong engine.

Back up. Restart the starboard. Shut down the **port**. Fortunately, just ahead was a small bay. I eased us in, dropped a short anchor, and cut the starboard engine.

"Just Breathe," I told myself.

I climbed back down, threw an old blanket over the oily mess on the floor, and carefully lowered myself into the engine compartment.

It didn't take long to spot the problem: the oil cap on the port engine was missing. Oil had sprayed out like a firehose, coating the engine room and half the starboard engine.

To this day, I don't know exactly what happened. Maybe I forgot to put the cap on after checking the oil that morning. Maybe I didn't seat it properly and it worked itself loose.

Either way, the damage wasn't just mechanical—it was emotional. It would take me weeks to fully clean that mess.

The immediate concern: *Was the engine damaged?* The urgent problem: *We didn't have enough oil on board to refill the reservoir.*

Let me pause the story here and own something hard: I wasn't prepared. Not really. I had checked the oil, sure—but I didn't carry nearly enough onboard to handle a full refill. It wasn't on my radar, and that's on me.

From that day forward, I made sure we had enough oil to change out an entire engine. I never needed it again—but I slept better knowing it was there.

Call it a lesson in humility, or just the old Boy Scout motto catching up with me: Be prepared.

Be Prepared (or Else)

And here's another Loop truth the day drove home: consequences still exist.

You can't loophole your way around them out here. There's no principal's office or customer service line. If something goes wrong on your boat, it's yours to fix.

Every misstep, every drop of oil in the bilge, it was all on me. And weirdly enough, that kind of ownership felt... good. Grounding. Like I'd crossed an invisible threshold in seamanship—and maybe in life.

It's a hard-earned lesson we don't teach often enough anymore.

The Trouble with Trophies

I want to say this gently, but with conviction: we've grown soft as a society. Somewhere along the way, in our well-meaning attempt to protect feelings and build self-esteem, we embraced the "everyone gets a trophy" mindset.

At first glance, it seemed like a kindness—a way to make every child feel like a winner. But in doing so, we unintentionally stripped away something far more valuable than temporary affirmation: we lost the gift of earned success.

I didn't grow up in that world. My trophies came with sweat and splinters. You earned your way to the podium—or you didn't. And if you didn't, you learned something, got better, and tried again.

Failure either made you grow, or look elsewhere for your place in the world. Not everyone is an NFL quarterback.

That cycle—of effort, failure, reevaluation, and eventual reward—wasn't easy, but it was real. And it stuck with you.

True confidence doesn't come from being handed a ribbon—it comes from facing challenges, learning through failure, and discovering that you're capable of more than you thought.

Struggle builds resilience. Disappointment teaches perspective. And effort, not entitlement, is what forges character.

By removing the natural tension between effort and reward, we diluted the lessons that once shaped strong, grounded, and capable individuals.

Growth was sacrificed for comfort.

Accountability took a back seat to affirmation.

In the process, we've raised a generation less prepared for the real world.

It's time we revisit the value of grit, personal responsibility, and the quiet strength that comes from earning—not being given—your place in the world.

Even though I never consciously subscribed to that "everyone gets a trophy" philosophy, I now realize that comfort had quietly crept into my life.

Over time, I had settled into a world I understood, a routine where I felt competent and in control. But in that comfort, I stopped noticing how much I didn't know.

I had become so secure in my own domain that I forgot what it felt like to be truly challenged.

The Loop changed that. It forced me to confront not just the unknown waters ahead, but also the blind spots within myself.

Time and again, I came face-to-face with situations that exposed how often I had leaned on other people's strengths—delegating, outsourcing, or simply avoiding what I didn't know how to do.

That might have worked on land. But on the Loop, when the wind picks up or the engine sputters, there's no one to call. It's just you and the moment.

Cruising those miles returned me to something essential: self-awareness.

I rediscovered my limits and my failures, but also my capacity to grow, adapt, and persevere. I remembered the quiet confidence that comes not from avoiding hard things, but from facing them head-on and figuring them out.

The Loop rekindled my belief in self-reliance and the deep, sustaining reward that comes from standing on your own two feet, especially when the dock is miles behind you.

But insights don't fix logistics. We still had a mess to deal with.

Operation Oil Run

Joanne started calling every nearby marina. None could take us in. Running on one engine wasn't a great option—not in these busy waters, with my limited experience.

I checked Google Maps and found the nearest auto parts store. The only way to get there was to dinghy to the nearest dock.

Of course, the dinghy had issues. I didn't realize at the time that the gas cap had to be loosened slightly for it to run properly. So every few minutes, it died. Doug and Jana stayed aboard while Joanne and I limped to a private dock at a nearby high-rise condo complex.

I ran off to meet our Uber driver, leaving Joanne behind.

Almost immediately, a security guard showed up. Joanne, in classic fashion, told him the whole story—tears and all. He let her stay, though he kept circling back every fifteen minutes, probably expecting her to flee the scene.

Meanwhile, I was in an Uber with a driver who didn't speak English. Thank God for the Google Translate app. We made it work. We got the oil.

I ended up having to pay him cash to hang around while I picked up the oil. Of course, all I had was a $100 bill, and he conveniently had no change.

Back at the dock, Joanne nearly cried with relief. We loaded the oil into the dinghy, crossed our fingers, and pushed off—hoping the motor would cooperate for the half-mile trip back to the boat.

It didn't. The engine died every 50 yards.

The rhythm was absurd: sputter, stall, row, repeat. After 15 minutes of stop-and-go effort, arms aching and patience thinning, we finally reached the swim platform.

But the work wasn't over.

I climbed aboard, poured in the oil, and whispered a prayer as I turned the key.

Return to Calm

The engine started.

It ran like nothing had ever gone wrong—no knocking, no smoke, just the familiar hum of a healthy engine. Later, oil analysis confirmed what I'd hoped: no damage.

By the grace of God, I had shut it down just in time. And for the record—not a single drop of oil left the boat. The spill was fully contained in the bilge, as designed.

Here's the kicker.

That night at anchor in Hollywood Beach, the sunset was outrageous—orange and pink and everything in between. There's a photo of Joanne and me on the swim deck, soaking it in. We look relaxed, happy, like it was just another perfect day on the Loop.

There's not a trace of panic on my face. And that, my friend, is the art of Looping.

What I Learned from the Spill

Looking back, the Great Oil Spill wasn't just a mess to clean up—it was a mirror. It reflected how quickly things can unravel, how unprepared I still was, and how grace can arrive in surprising forms: a flash of awareness, a steady partner, and an engine willing to forgive your mistakes.

I learned that cruising life isn't just about weather forecasts and fuel gauges. It's about how you handle the unexpected. About staying calm when everything in you wants to panic. About laughing later at what nearly unraveled you in the moment.

And maybe most of all, I learned that some of the best sunsets come after the worst days—when you've been humbled, stretched, and somehow made it through.

LOOP LESSONS: THE GREAT OIL SPILL

Even seasoned routines need a double-check. Complacency causes more problems than inexperience—always double-check the basics, even if you've done them a hundred times.

Panic is a poor mechanic. When stress spikes, slow down. Clarity comes from calm, not chaos.

Every crisis is a character test. The way you handle a setback reveals more about you than the setback itself.

The dinghy has opinions of its own. Know your tender as well as your trawler—it's your lifeline more often than you think.

You can't plan every problem, but you can prepare your mindset. Flexibility, humility, and humor go farther than any spare part.

Setbacks don't cancel beauty. A day that starts in panic can still end in peace—with a killer sunset and a sense of perspective.

Tell the story. Even your worst moments on the Loop become part of the tapestry. If you're still afloat, it's a good story.

Self-reliance is earned, not assumed. On the water, there's no one to bail you out. You either solve the problem or drift with it. The Loop forces you to become your own mechanic, planner, and emergency responder.

Own your mistakes. The oil spill was my fault. But taking responsibility was a turning point. Blame doesn't fix a bilge full of oil. Action does.

Emotional resilience matters as much as mechanical skill. A calm mind and a steady hand often solve more problems than tools or tech. When things go sideways, breathe first. Then act.

Laugh when you can—even if it's later. Humor doesn't erase the chaos, but it softens it. Looking back, rowing a dying dinghy every 50 yards was ridiculous... and kind of perfect.

The Loop doesn't just show you the world—it shows you yourself. It's a mirror. A teacher. A test. And sometimes, a gentle rebuke with a beautiful reward.

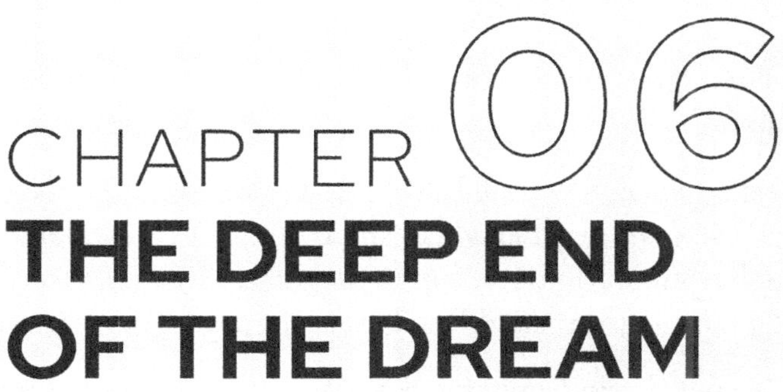

CHAPTER 06
THE DEEP END OF THE DREAM

Conversation in Charleston

April 19-- I didn't know it at the time, but a quiet conversation on a dock in Charleston would become one of the defining moments of my Loop.

"You look relaxed," the passerby said, eyeing the AGLCA flag flying from our boat. "I've always wanted to do that trip. How long have you been on the Loop?"

He lingered for a moment, clearly curious. "So... how's it going? What's it been like?"

I smiled, took a slow breath, and replied, "It's more than I ever imagined it would be."

We were in Charleston, South Carolina, some 1,500 miles into the trip, and things were finally starting to make sense. My wife, Joanne, and I hadn't exactly taken to cruising easily.

The learning curve had been steep for both of us—full of unknowns, and more than a few humbling moments. But we were finding our footing.

We were settling into a rhythm that felt more like home. And it wasn't until this tourist struck up a conversation, pressing me to put the experience into words, that I realized just how much we were both changing.

I don't remember exactly how I worded it, but I hope it sounded something like this:

"Friend, sitting here, right now—a cold drink in my hand, on the bow of my own boat, just me and my thoughts—the trip has been awesome, but I've been through a few storms. You can probably tell. It's in the worn creases of my shirt, in the way my shoulders don't carry urgency anymore.

I'm not in a rush. I'm not chasing anything these days. I'm not sitting here replaying all the moments I got it wrong. I'm thinking about how right it feels to finally just sit still, to breathe without bracing for what's next."

"That look in my eye? It's relief. Relief that I came out the other side of those first days on the Loop, the ones where every moment was full of the unknown. Now? I've found peace—not in noise or motion, but in the quiet. In the satisfaction of this boat being my home. In the steady rhythm of waves breaking just beyond the rocks, out of sight but always there."

Like so many I'd meet along the way, this man wasn't just curious—he was yearning.

Not jealous, exactly, but searching. There was a quiet hurt in his voice, a look in his eyes I knew all too well.

He was adrift, and he sensed that maybe—just maybe—I'd found the course he'd been trying to chart.

I had been that man. Same eyes. Same questions. Same longing. Same lostness. And in that moment, I wanted more than anything to help him find his way.

"Man," he said, half-smiling, "I've been watching YouTube videos and reading everything I can about the Loop. It just looks... awesome. Maybe someday..."

His voice faded, but his eyes drifted to some distant place only he could see—already aboard his own boat, casting off lines, leaving the noise behind. I knew that feeling.

Been there, done that

I'd spent years walking docks, scanning for Looper flags, hoping for a conversation like the one we were now having.

Hoping for someone to tell me it wasn't impossible. So I gave him the words I once longed to hear:

"I'm not lost anymore. I'm just far enough from the noise now to actually hear myself again.

Maybe you're not here yet. Maybe you're still caught in your storm, trying to find your way through. But I promise you—stillness is real. It's out there, waiting. And one day, you'll find yourself right where I am."

Leaning back, sipping slow, and smiling because you found your way home too.

Truth is, I'm sure I didn't say it nearly as eloquently back then—but 4,500 cruising miles later, I've had time to shape the words and sharpen the insight. What I now understand, I've earned through experience.

The Pull of The Water

I've always been drawn to the water, but that connection has only deepened over time. I can lose myself for hours just watching the ocean, mesmerized by the rhythm of the waves.

One of the biggest reasons the Loop captivated me was the opportunity to live ***on*** the water—not just beside it. It didn't disappoint.

The water became my moat, putting space between me and the demands of everyday life. It didn't shield me from everything, but it did provide a much-needed buffer—a quiet, welcome distance from the noise of the real world.

My favorite artist, Kenny Chesney, has built an entire career around the truth that water isn't just a setting—it's an escape. He doesn't just sing about the sea; he lives it.

When he's not on tour, you'll often find him tucked away in the Virgin Islands, where the salt air and slow pace offer him both creativity and renewal. It's not just his backdrop—it's his way back to himself.

It wasn't until we were deep into the Loop, somewhere quiet and still, that I started to experience what he sings about.

As Kenny Chesney said in an American Songwriter interview in 2018, "I've always been drawn to the ocean." That's not just a lyric—it's a knowing. A kind of soul recognition.

During the year aboard PATIENCE, I came to learn what Chesney often tells his fans: "Time spent on the water is never wasted." It's not an escape—it's a return. To yourself. To rhythm. To the version of you that isn't performing or producing or planning. The version of you that just is.

There was one morning in particular in Georgia, at a favorite Looper stop, Sunbury Crab Company—early light, glassy calm—when I sat on the aft deck with my coffee, no agenda, no hurry. And in that stillness, I felt it.

"When I look out into the ocean," Chesney once said, "it reminds me of how infinite our possibilities are. The ocean really humbles me." I knew exactly what he meant. Out there, life doesn't feel small—but it does feel right-sized.

We weathered some storms along the way—both on the water and within.

At times I felt unsure, overwhelmed, and completely out of my depth. But the heart of songs like *Better Boat*—about letting go, adapting, and learning through hardship—stopped feeling like lyrics and started feeling like lived experience. It became my truth.

You don't finish the Loop the same person you were when you cast off the lines. You get reshaped by the water—softened, steadied, and made new.

There's no applause out there. No spotlight. Just the slow, quiet work of transformation.

And for me, it started when I realized the water wasn't just scenery. It was sanctuary.

Blue Mind

I only recently learned there's a name for this phenomenon: Blue Mind. Popularized by marine biologist Dr. Wallace J. Nichols, the Blue Mind theory describes the mildly meditative state we enter when we're near or around water. And I absolutely believe it.

Whether I'm beside the ocean, floating on a lake, swimming in a river, or even soaking in a hot tub, I feel more relaxed, inspired, and at ease.

I've discovered that water doesn't just affect how I feel—it actually changes what's happening in my body and brain.

It boosts my well-being by increasing the levels of dopamine (the feel-good hormone), serotonin (the happiness hormone), and oxytocin (the cuddle hormone), while lowering cortisol, the stress hormone.

When I'm around water, something shifts in my attention. My brain relaxes and opens up, and I find it easier to solve problems and think creatively. Water seems to invite awe—and in doing so, it also deepens my sense of compassion and connection to others.

Even just the sight, sound, or feel of water can lower my heart rate and help me feel grounded.

That's the power of Blue Mind, and it's become something I turn to whenever I need to reset, reflect, or simply breathe.

I know you didn't pick up this book for a science lesson—but trust me, spending a few minutes understanding the idea behind Blue Mind will deepen everything that follows. It's the lens through which much of this journey—and its impact—makes sense.

RED MIND -VS- BLUE MIND

Dr. Wallace J. Nichols' book Blue Mind (2014) contrasts the stress-driven, "always-on" Red Mind—characterized by anxiety, overstimulation, and elevated stress hormones—with the calmer, more centered Blue Mind, which is associated with being immersed in or near water, mindfulness, and reduced physiological stress.

He charts it in an effective way that allows us to see the difference:

● Red Mind vs. ● **Blue Mind**

● Red Mind

Category:

Emotional State. Anxious, irritable, overstimulated.

Triggers. Deadlines, screens, noise.

Physiological. Elevated cortisol and adrenaline.

Mental Focus. Scattered, reactive

Health Impact. Burnout, sleep issues, chronic stress.

● Blue Mind

Emotional State.. Calm, reflective, centered

Triggers. . Nature, water, quiet, mindfulness

Physiological. Lower heart rate, reduced stress hormones

Mental Focus Focused, creative, present

Health Impact. Improved well-being, clarity,

Nichols' "Red Mind vs. Blue Mind" chart offers a clear snapshot of a deeper truth: modern life wears us down, but water has the power to restore us. His work draws from the broader science of *blue space* and *biophilia*—the innate human pull toward nature.

Biologist Edward O. Wilson, in *Biophilia* (1984), put it simply: we're wired to seek out life. And water, more than almost anything else, activates that connection—triggering real, measurable benefits for both body and mind.

Modern research supports this ancient connection. In two studies, researchers found that simply looking at water can significantly reduce stress.

In one experiment, participants who gazed at a swimming pool for just 100 seconds showed lower blood pressure and heart rate than those who looked at a tree or a street sign.

A larger study in a university arboretum echoed earlier findings: participants had lower heart rates and blood pressure when viewing lakes and a creek versus grassy or wooded areas.

The results suggest we're hardwired for calm near water—confirming the relaxation many feel isn't just in our heads (White, Gatersleben, & Pahl, 2010).

The work of Wilson and Nichols reinforces this: time spent near water—or in a Blue Mind state—can counteract the stress of our hyper-connected, fast-paced Red Mind lives.

This insight now shapes conversations around mental health, biophilia, and nature-based healing.

I'm not trying to dive too deep into psychology, but it's clear to me now that what I experienced on the Loop wasn't just personal preference—it was something deeper.

For years, I couldn't explain my pull toward the water. Now I see it's rooted in something fundamental, even biological. Spending a year on the Loop slowed me down, helped me see problems in perspective, and made me feel fully alive.

These days, I don't just enjoy the water—I intentionally pursue a Blue Mind way of life.

I've lost count of the moments on the Loop that confirm this truth.

One of the most unforgettable came as we neared the end of our journey, anchored on the quiet waters of the Tensaw River. We were about 150 miles from crossing our wake. It was November 6th, my 63rd birthday, but it felt like I was in another world.

That day, we cruised 83 miles alongside the boat, Valkyrie, who dropped anchor about 500 yards from us. We grilled a couple of steaks, poured some wine, and simply soaked in the moment.

The sunset—pure magic—was nature's gift that night. You can see it on our Facebook page, "Loop of Faith." Honestly, it was one of the greatest nights of my life. That was one of the Loop's gifts to me.

How to Apply Blue Mind Daily

After completing the Loop and returning to dirt life, Joanne and I incorporated Blue Mind into our daily lives. Some of these are more for her than me, but they all make life better:

* Go there physically: swim, paddle, walk along a creek, sit by a fountain.

* Bring it home: take mindful baths, install small water features, use recordings or imagery.

* Try a retreat: book a spa day, take a therapeutic boat ride, or plan a minimal-technology getaway near water.

* Micro doses: just spending two minutes watching waves or running water can reset your nervous system.

The Great Loop didn't just take me around the eastern half of the country; it brought me inward, into stillness, into clarity, into peace. I set out chasing adventure and found transformation. Water was the vehicle, the teacher, and the sanctuary.

And now I know this for sure: the calm we crave isn't out there somewhere—it's in us, waiting to be uncovered.

Sometimes, it just takes 6,000 miles of waves to hear what your soul's been whispering all along.

LOOP LESSONS FROM THE DEEP END OF THE DREAM:

Water isn't scenery; it's sanctuary. Living *on* the water creates a buffer from everyday demands and invites deep restoration.

Time on the water is never wasted—it's a return to self. It strips away performance mode and reconnects you with who you are beneath the to-do lists.

Perspective expands at the shoreline. Vast horizons humble you and right-size life's problems.

Storms teach seamanship of the soul. Riding out literal and figurative waves fosters resilience—"building a better boat" within.

Transformation happens quietly, without applause. Long stretches of stillness do the slow work of reshaping character.

"Blue Mind" is real biology, not poetry. Proximity to water raises dopamine, serotonin, and oxytocin while lowering cortisol.

Creativity and problem-solving flourish near water. A calm brain becomes an open, imaginative brain.

Blue Mind counteracts "Red Mind." Water's calm neutralizes the anxiety, overstimulation, and elevated stress hormones of modern life.

Humans are wired for blue spaces. Studies show heart rate and blood pressure drop within seconds of watching water.

Anchored moments become touchstones. A sunset on the Tensaw River or dawn coffee at Sunbury Crab Company can mark life's highlight reel.

Micro-doses work. Two minutes of watching or listening to water can reset the nervous system.

Bring Blue Mind home. Fountains, a dip in a pool, and water sounds let you tap its benefits even on land.

Stillness is the destination. Getting far enough from the noise lets you finally hear yourself again.

Return to Blue Mind when life gets loud. It's the quickest path back to calm, clarity, and your best self.

CHAPTER 07
THE CREWS THAT CARRIED US

Most books and YouTube channels about the Great Loop focus on the journey itself—the routes, the marinas, the sights, and the stats.

And while all of that is part of the magic, don't miss what I believe is the true heart of the experience, and what will live the longest after you cross your wake: the people.

There's simply no better part of the Loop than the friendships you form along the way. Other than my church family, the Looper community is unlike anything I've ever been part of—welcoming, generous, wise, and deeply supportive.

I honestly don't think we could have completed the journey without them. Time and again, I leaned on fellow Loopers—for advice, encouragement, a helping hand, or just a voice on the radio when things got tough.

Many of the most important lessons I learned out there didn't come from the charts or cruising guides—they came from the people. Their kindness, example, and quiet wisdom shaped me just as much as the miles did. This chapter is about them.

MIKE AND GRAYCE- The Ones Who Went Before

We met Mike and Grayce right after they finished their Loop aboard *Grayceful Waterbug*—the boat we would purchase and rename *PATIENCE.*

I had been searching for a Loop boat for months. I even had one surveyed, only to walk away when engine issues surfaced. But when I found PATIENCE, I knew. She wasn't just the right boat—she was the one.

I truly believe we ended up with the boat God intended for us to have. She fit us perfectly and carried us nearly 6,000 miles with remarkable grace and reliability.

Finding PATIENCE was no accident.

We first spotted her on the AGLCA Facebook page—a post that felt more like divine appointment than coincidence. Kim Russo and her team at the AGLCA do incredible work, offering a wide range of support to Loopers at every stage of the journey.

Like many others, we were guided early on by the AGLCA's resources and community. Their website, in-person events, and network of Harbor Hosts formed a kind of invisible safety net that gave us the confidence to move forward—especially in those uncertain first weeks.

I highly recommend joining the Association if you want to learn about the Loop.

From my first conversation with Mike H., I could tell he was the real deal—honest, kind, and wired to help others. He had a wealth of knowledge about boats in general, and about PATIENCE in particular.

He'd put in countless upgrades and had her systems dialed in, ready to go. Good thing, too—because we pulled away from the dock just three days after signing the papers.

Mike and Grayce spent two full days on board with us, walking us through the systems, answering every question, and giving us enough confidence to at least pretend we knew what we were doing.

Those two days were invaluable—not just because of what we learned, but because we saw ourselves in them.

They were experienced boaters—especially Mike, who came from a competitive sailing background—but even so, this type of cruising was new to them. It was reassuring to hear Grayce say, with such calm certainty, "You can do it. Just give it three months. It'll start to feel natural."

And she was right. Almost to the day, three months in, we finally felt like we had found our rhythm.

But I won't lie—those first three months were hard. Really hard. There were moments when I genuinely questioned whether we had made a mistake. The steep learning curve was stealing the joy and turning the dream into a burden.

Grayce, if you ever read this—thank you. Your words in Destin stayed with us. Without them, we might have given up.

I remember one night at a lonely anchorage outside Cape Canaveral, Joanne and I sat on the aft deck, worn out and worn down. We had a raw, honest conversation about what we had signed up for and where we really were, both emotionally and mentally. We had come to the edge.

We had to ask the question neither of us wanted to say out loud: "Do we keep going, or do we quit?"

That conversation didn't end the Loop—but it reshaped it. It reminded us why we started, and what we still hoped to find out there. And looking back now, I'm so glad we kept going.

It became clear that it wasn't just Mike and Grayce's words that encouraged us—it was the example they set with every mile they'd already traveled. Only later did I understand how powerful that example really was.

One important lesson from that moment on the Atlantic Coast was this: words matter.

Your words of encouragement can have a lasting impact. Be mindful of what you say to others—and just as importantly, of the words you choose to receive—because they carry the power to shape lives, steer decisions, and change someone's course entirely.

The right words can steady you—but sometimes, it's the right people who carry you the rest of the way. That's what happened next.

Chad and Nancy *(Soul of a Sailor)*--**Brotherhood at Sea**

April 23 turned out to be a big day—though we didn't know it at the time.

We had just wrapped up six memorable days in Charleston, South Carolina. Joanne's brother, Jim, and his wife Selina had driven in from Tennessee to visit.

It felt good to share our journey with them—so much had already happened, and we were brimming with stories. Their visit gave us a chance to relive the adventure so far through fresh eyes.

But the Loop, as always, demanded our attention.

While in Charleston, we learned that a bridge ahead on the waterway—the Onslow Beach Bridge at Mile Marker 240—was about reportedly going to close for almost a month due to repairs.

That gave us just four days to cover 216 miles or risk being stranded south of the bridge till it reopened.

The clock was ticking.

Joanne sprang into action, rescheduling marina stops and rerouting our plans. It meant skipping a few places we'd been looking forward to, but suddenly, what had been a leisurely coastal run turned into a race against time.

As we departed Charleston that morning, a loose procession of a dozen Loopers began making their way out as well, leaving from different marinas but all heading the same direction.

We found ourselves tucked in just behind another Silverton yacht—SOUL OF A SAILOR.

We'd briefly encountered them way back in Florida, at Lighthouse Point Marina in Pompano Beach. They had just returned from the Bahamas and were refueling to head out again.

Joanne met Nancy on the dock and exchanged boat cards while her husband, Chad, wrapped up fueling. The whole interaction lasted less than five minutes—just a passing moment.

What we didn't know then was that those five minutes were the beginning of something special. Before long, SOUL OF A SAILOR and its crew would feel more like family than fellow travelers.

Chad and Nancy were both recently retired from the Navy, where they had met, married, and raised a family of 2 daughters.

The Loop was their reward—a way to celebrate the close of one chapter and reset their lives to a new rhythm.

Chad had served as a Navy diver, a skill that came in handy more than once on the Loop. He was a true MacGyver—give him a roll of tape and a paper clip, and he could fix just about anything.

Nancy had worked in IT, but it didn't take long to sense that she was glad to have left that world behind. Out here, she seemed light, at ease—ready for something slower and grounded.

Chad and Nancy handled their 43-foot yacht with such ease, it was like watching seasoned pros at work. Every docking, every departure—they made it look effortless.

Joanne and I couldn't help but feel a little envious, and even more determined to reach that level of confidence ourselves.

From the beginning, it felt like a friendship that was meant to happen. Both of us owned Silvertons—theirs a 43MY ours a 39MY—but aside from a few feet of length and an extra foot of beam, the boats were nearly twins.

And the similarities didn't stop there. We each had two daughters, good marriages and a love of adventure.

Chad and I hit it off right away.

Despite being more than a decade apart in age, we were both born in November—just one day apart. As Scorpios, we were almost too similar: driven, intense, and always chasing the next adventure.

We shared a love for music, boats, fishing, golf, and squeezing the most out of life.

I can say without hesitation that if it weren't for the Loop, our paths never would've crossed.

Looking back, I realized something surprising—since high school, every close friend I'd made had come through either church or work.

Chad was different. He didn't fit any of the usual categories. He was like me... but not. He grew up on the shores of the Chesapeake in Maryland; I came up on ranches and farms in California.

Our worlds couldn't have been more different, and yet we found an easy rhythm together.

The Loop cut new paths *through* me in ways I didn't expect—especially when it came to relationships. It broke me out of the narrow lanes I'd traveled for years and showed me the richness that comes from connecting with people whose lives looked nothing like mine.

Chad was a perfect example. Our backgrounds were worlds apart, but somehow, out on the water, those differences didn't divide us—they deepened the friendship.

The Loop broadened my view of people and deepened my appreciation for the rich variety God created.

After traveling together that first day, we shared docktails and agreed to follow the same route up to Onslow Bridge. What started as a short-term plan turned into many miles of shared waters over the course of the journey.

Chad and Nancy approached the Loop with military-like precision and discipline.

Watching them showed me that the Loop demanded that kind of attention to detail.

From maintenance schedules to route planning to weather checks—everything had to be handled as if our lives depended on it. Because, in truth, they did.

In the end, we logged over 2,900 miles together.

Soul of a Sailor became our trusted "buddy boat," and we now have thousands of photos capturing our two vessels side by side in some of the most stunning ports in the world. Check it out on our Facebook page, *"Loop of Faith"*.

Getting to know people from such different backgrounds opened my eyes to whole new ways of living. Hearing their stories and seeing the world through their lens was both refreshing and inspiring—one more insight the Loop uncovered along the way.

By the end of our journey, we had a small business-card box overflowing with boat cards—custom cards that Loopers exchange, usually featuring their boat name, crew names, hailing port, and contact info.

Each one was a reminder of someone we met, each representing a fresh perspective and a unique outlook on life.

Connecting with new people quickly became one of my favorite parts of the Loop.

It also taught me to lift my eyes, to be more present and open to those around me. Slowing down long enough to truly get to know others expanded my world in ways I didn't expect. It made me more inclusive, more aware, and more curious.

By listening to how others see the world, I found my own vision stretching. I didn't realize how much I needed that.

I expect we would have made it around the Loop without Chad and Nancy—after all, we did half of it on our own. But I can say this with certainty: I became a better captain, and a more well-rounded person, because they became our friends.

For the rest of my life, whenever I hear Kenny Chesney sing, "*Soul of a Sailor*" I'll be swept back into the tide of the Loop—and find myself right there with you.

Thank you, both—you made the journey richer.

The Loop never failed to deliver unforgettable people—this time in the form of joy, laughter, and a spontaneous cannonball into the bay.

Mike and Pam (*Thyme Away*) --The Joyful Cannonball

We first met Mike and Pam (Thyme Away) at Frying Pan Bay, a beloved anchorage nestled in Canada's Georgian Bay—one of the most breathtaking spots on the entire Loop. We had docked side by side, surrounded by a cluster of other boats.

The scene was pure joy: paddle boards gliding by, fishing lines cast lazily into the water, kids laughing from floats, and everyone soaking in the magic of the moment.

Mike carried the same sense of wonder I felt when we first started. They were just beginning their Loop, while we were already 3,300 miles into ours.

Mike was full of questions—soaking up every bit of advice I could offer with genuine excitement. He was a joy to be around—always smiling, always warm, and always up for a good conversation.

Mike reminded me that it takes no more energy to be joyful than it does to be miserable.

The first moment I saw him is etched in my memory—Mike, grinning ear to ear, leapt off the bow of his boat to join a group of kids splashing in the water.

Their laughter echoed through the bay, and Mike laughed the loudest of all. The kids adored him—and honestly, so did everyone else.

That moment left a mark: I want to live more like that—open, joyful, and more in awe of life.

As Kenny Chesney sings, you only get *"one ticket to the big dance"*—so you'd better make it count. Laugh loud, dance freely, chase the sunset, and live wide open—while you still can.

Not all bonds were formed by logging miles together—some Loopers made their mark simply by showing up, again and again, with spirit and heart

David and Tonya (*Pokey*) --Bold in a Small Boat

We first met David and Tonya on their boat, POKEY, on April 26 in Southport, South Carolina.

Our boat was docked just behind theirs, and I was immediately intrigued by their vessel—a small, custom-built boat powered by an outboard motor. It looked efficient and compact, but certainly not what I expected to see flying the AGLCA burgee.

That surprise only grew when the cabin door opened and out came the whole crew—David, Tonya, and their three dogs. "Wow," I said as we shook hands. "How far into the Loop are you?"

Turns out, they were already halfway through the journey, having completed some of the most challenging stretches, including the Gulf crossing. Because of their boat's size and low freeboard, they'd hugged the shoreline most of the way, carefully navigating with intention and grit.

There was no question their boat was capable—it had already proven itself—but I still couldn't believe it. I remember thinking, *This might be one of the most courageous crews I've ever met.*

I wouldn't have attempted the Loop in a boat that small, but David was a skilled captain, and he approached the voyage with a calm confidence that earned my respect.

We leapfrogged (Loopers call it "Loop-frogging") with them up the East Coast, often spotting their boat anchored in quiet coves while we opted for marinas.

Anchoring not only saved them money—it was something they genuinely preferred.

They were doing the Loop frugally and intentionally—and doing it well. We shared a few dinners along the way, including one in Belhaven, North Carolina, and another at the Solomons Yacht Club on the Chesapeake. We always enjoyed our time with them.

David was working nearly full-time during the trip, staying connected via Starlink. It was impressive—he kept pace with both his job and the journey, making it all look seamless.

David and Tonya embodied one of my favorite truths: **where there's a will, there's a way**.

I've met so many people who say they'll do the Loop "someday"—when they retire, when life slows down, when the stars align. But most never will.

David and Tonya didn't wait. They chose now. Their story reminds me that boldness often trumps perfection, and that sometimes the smallest boats carry the biggest dreams.

Looking back, I see now that the true course of the Great Loop isn't just plotted on charts—it's traced in conversations, laughter, shared sunsets, borrowed tools, and unexpected dockside moments.

These people weren't just fellow travelers; they became co-authors of our journey, shaping it in ways no itinerary ever could.

I set out chasing the adventure of a lifetime, but what I found was something even greater: a floating fellowship of souls who reminded me that we are meant to do life together.

None of this would've happened without the connective thread of the AGLCA. From the very start, their resources, events, and Harbor Hosts helped build the framework for these relationships to form.

More than just an organization, they created a space where strangers could become friends, where shared experience turned into lasting connection. In many ways, the AGLCA isn't just about navigation—it's about community. And for us, that community made all the difference.

If the Loop taught me anything, it's this—beautiful places will stir your spirit, but it's the people who change your life.

LOOP LESSONS FROM "THE PEOPLE WHO MADE THE LOOP"

People are the heart of the Loop. The journey is memorable, but the relationships are what leave a lasting imprint.

Community is stronger than charts. The advice, kindness, and support of fellow Loopers often proved more valuable than any cruising guide.

Mentors matter. Seasoned Loopers like Mike and Grayce helped us begin with confidence and reminded us to hang in through the hard parts.

Encouraging words stick. A single, well-timed "You can do it" can keep someone from giving up. Speak them generously.

Shared miles create deep bonds. Traveling with others—like Chad and Nancy on SOUL OF A SAILOR—transforms strangers into family.

Friendship knows no background. The Loop brings together people from wildly different walks of life and proves how much we all share.

The Loop widens your lens. Hearing how others live, think, and see the world expands your empathy and curiosity.

Excellence is contagious. Watching detail-oriented boaters sharpened our own discipline and seamanship.

Joy is magnetic. People like Mike on THYME AWAY reminded us that choosing joy is often just that—a choice.

Boldness over perfection. David and Tonya on POKEY showed that you don't need a big boat or perfect timing—just the will to go.

Loopers live out loud. Whether it's laughter in a quiet anchorage or a leap into new friendships, the Loop encourages wholehearted living.

You become who you cruise with. The people you surround yourself with influence how you experience the journey—and who you become along the way.

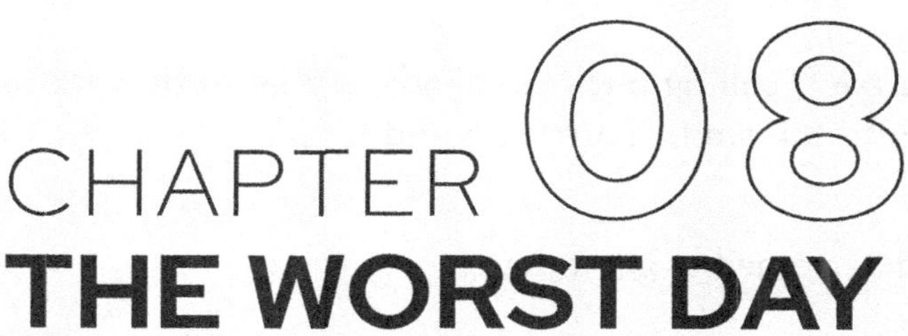

CHAPTER 08
THE WORST DAY

July 1 might've been the worst day of our entire Loop.

We were on the Erie Canal, facing seven locks—the most we'd ever attempted in a single stretch—and nearly everything that could go wrong... did.

But it wasn't just the mechanical stress or the surprises in the water. What made it *the worst* was how close we came to disaster—on every front.

Boiling Waters, Boiling Tempers

It all started at the second lock of the day. The lockmaster radioed that they were making repairs and asked us to tie up along the approach wall, just short of the chamber.

I was already close to the entrance, so I tried to simply slide over and tie off on the starboard side.

I should've known better.

The current near the lock entrance suddenly started boiling and swirling in unpredictable patterns. It seized PATIENCE like a toy, yanking her bow and slamming her rub rail against the concrete wall. I had almost no control.

I tried to ease her against the wall, but it towered above our bow rail, and the turbulence made it nearly impossible to hold position.

Joanne scrambled forward and began trying to lasso a bollard nearly four feet away.

I was already on edge, calling out commands, trying to prevent us from slamming into the wall. "Hurry up and tie off!" I barked. "I can't hold her!"

Jo kept trying—determined to get it done.

Then she made a dangerous move. She later told me she never felt at risk—she felt in control. But from where I stood, it was a different story.

Under pressure, she placed one foot on the wall and tried to straddle the gap between boat and concrete. She was just trying to do her job—trying to keep the boat safe.

For one gut-wrenching moment, she was caught between them—half in, half out—suspended between fiberglass and concrete.

I was livid.

"Get on the boat!" I shouted. She hesitated.

"Get on the boat!" Louder.

"GET ON THE BOAT!" The words ricocheted off the walls of the lock approach.

Determination burned in her eyes as she finally lassoed the bollard and stepped back aboard. She moved aft in silence.

When the chaos finally settled, I turned to her, my voice cracking.

"I had almost no control in that current," I said quietly. "If you'd slipped—even with your PFD—you could've been crushed between the boat and the wall."

"I didn't think of that" she said.

She could've died. I wasn't angry. I was scared to death.

Our buddy boat, *Annie Marie,* had been right behind us. Mark and Terry saw the whole thing unfold.

That evening, over a quiet dinner on the banks of the Erie, they gently reinforced what I'd said.

"That was a dangerous thing to do," Mark said. "Please don't do it again."

It makes for a good story now.

But in the moment? It was terrifying.

Mistakes Compound

But the day wasn't finished with us.

At the very next lock, just as we were easing back into the canal, the radio crackled.

"Hey, *PATIENCE*, you've got a line in the water."

I looked aft and felt my stomach drop. One of our mooring lines was dragging alongside the boat like a sea serpent, weaving in and out of the wake.

"What? I had all of them secured," Jo said, frustrated.

"Apparently not," I quipped. "Hurry and get it out of the water—I'll hold steady."

It had slipped overboard, unnoticed.

"That seems about par for the day," I muttered, knowing it probably didn't help.

"Careful there, Captain," she shot back. "It hasn't been your best day either."

Of course, she was right.

It was a simple mistake—one anyone could make after seven exhausting locks and a morning full of tension. But in that moment, it felt like the kind of slip that could wreck your whole day—or worse, your boat.

If I'd backed down or turned too sharply, that line could've wrapped around the propeller shaft. One foul-up, and we'd be looking at a bent prop, a thrown shaft, or a costly haul-out.

No more words were exchanged as she reeled it back in—just the sight of rope against fiberglass and the steady thrum of the engines beneath our feet.

We were both worn out. Embarrassed. Frustrated.

That loose line felt like the perfect metaphor for the day: things unraveling, slipping just out of our control, barely holding it all together.

And still... the canal stretched ahead. More locks, more lessons. And a long way to go before sundown.

Autopilot Mayhem

At Lock 6, I made another mistake—one I still don't fully understand.

We had just finished locking up and I was easing us forward, ready to exit the chamber. Everything felt routine... until it didn't.

In hindsight, I must've accidentally nudged the autopilot button.

I don't use the wheel at slow speeds, preferring the throttles. But what I didn't realize was that the rudder was somehow turned hard to starboard.

So when I engaged the engines—boom. *PATIENCE* lunged to starboard like a spooked horse.

Jo was still on the bow, rolling up the lines. "What are you doing?" she yelled.

"I don't know what's going on," I snapped, wrestling with the throttles. "She won't respond."

In seconds, we were veering sideways—the bow cutting toward the right-hand wall while the stern swung left, scraping along the port-side concrete, with barely a boat length of room to recover.

For a terrifying moment, I thought we were going to hit the wall head-on.

"Watch out!" she warned.

"Doing the best I can," I fired back.

"The stern's about to hit the wall," she said.

Too late.

I adjusted the throttles and tried to correct, but not before the stern rub rail scraped hard against the lock wall.

The sound of grinding metal echoed off the chamber like a scream.

I imagined gouges, shattered gelcoat, and splintered panels.

But when I finally got control and eased her straight, I stepped back to inspect. No visible damage. Just the rub rail doing its job—taking the hit so the hull didn't have to.

Still, the noise alone rattled me.

In a day already full of emotional misfires and near-misses, this one shook my confidence all over again.

In hindsight, I must've accidentally nudged the autopilot button.

My mind was nearly cooked... and the day still wasn't done.

The Thump and the Vibration

Just when we thought the day couldn't throw anything else at us—it did.

After leaving Lock 6, cruising slow and steady through the canal, we hit something—hard. A deep, resonant *thump* echoed through the hull. It wasn't the kind of bump you dismiss.

"What was that?" Jo asked.

I looked over my shoulder and saw the top of a log roll to the surface. It had been hiding just below the waterline.

At first, everything seemed fine. The engines hummed. Steering responded.

"Maybe it's okay," I mumbled.

But after we exited Lock 7 and throttled up, the boat began to shudder.

"Great," I muttered. "Just what we need. Will this day never end?"

Not subtly—a deep, rhythmic vibration rolled through the deck like a warning bell. It was unmistakable... and unwelcome.

My heart sank.

In that moment, a mental slideshow played: bent shaft, damaged prop, haul-out, blown schedule, thousands in repairs. I felt the whole journey grind to a halt in my imagination.

I pulled back the throttles, trying to think clearly.

Then Jo, calmly and practically—because that's who she is—said: "Maybe something's just wrapped around the prop."

It stopped me. I stared ahead for a beat, then nodded. "Worth a try."

The locks and the canal were full of weeds and debris, so maybe...

I shifted into reverse, then throttled up both engines—hard—for about ten seconds. The stern kicked up a swirl of brown water, bits of vegetation flying out behind us.

Then I eased back into forward and brought the throttles up slowly.

The vibration was gone.

I let out a breath I hadn't realized I was holding.

It was weeds. Just weeds. Caught in the prop during that last lock. All that dread, all that mental spiraling—for a clump of greenery.

"Good call there," I said, letting some joy back into my voice. "Now let's get this boat to a dock and end this miserable day."

"I'm right there with you," Jo said with a sigh. "I'm exhausted."

But that's how it works on the Loop. One moment, you're imagining the worst. The next, you're moving forward again.

We laughed. Eventually.

But in the moment, it felt like one final test—one last gut punch from a day determined to humble us.

And it did.

A Day That Changed Us

There's no badge for surviving a day like that.

No trophy, no photo op, no pleasant memory. Just the quiet recognition that sometimes the Loop doesn't test your navigation—it tests your nerves, your marriage, your patience, your trust.

July 1 wasn't a day we'll ever brag about.

It won't make the highlight reel or get mentioned when people ask for our favorite moments on the Loop.

But that's the thing about transformative days—they're often the ones no one sees coming and no one would choose.

Looking back, that day didn't just reveal our limits. It revealed what grace looks like in a high-stakes, low-margin environment.

When everything was fraying, we had to decide whether we would fray too—or hold each other together.

We made mistakes—several of them.

Some were small, others could've cost us dearly.

But the Loop doesn't just teach you how to avoid error. It teaches you how to recover from it.

How to apologize without ego. How to lead without blame. How to protect each other, even when you're both worn thin.

That day demanded everything we had, and then some.

But we didn't break. We adjusted. We kept going.

And in the silence that followed—after the shouting, after the tension, after the fear—there was something else: a kind of quiet respect for what we'd endured, and a deeper trust that we'd face the next storm with more grace.

It was the worst day on the Loop.

But it may have been one of the most important.

Because it reminded us that resilience isn't proven on the good days. It's revealed in the hard ones.

LOOP LESSONS – THE WORST DAY

The Loop doesn't just test your seamanship—it tests your soul. The hardest days aren't always about mechanical failures or missed waypoints; they're about keeping your head and heart intact under pressure.

Grace matters most in the aftermath. Mistakes will happen. What defines you is how you respond—to yourself, to your partner, and to the moment.

A strong voice does not require a hard heart. Urgency can sound like anger in crisis, but often the loudest words are spoken out of deepest care.

Fatigue turns small errors into major events. Exhaustion dulls your edge, which is why grace—not perfection—must become the goal.

Danger rarely gives you advance notice. One misstep between fiberglass and concrete can change everything. Vigilance is not optional—it is essential.

Resilience is revealed in the recovery. What defines a journey is not the absence of failure, but the willingness to regroup and move forward.

Sometimes the best fix is a pause. One deep breath, one good idea, or one burst of reverse throttle can turn panic into progress.

Real partnership is forged in fire. Love deepens when it survives days like this—when connection wins out over criticism.

Not everything is as catastrophic as it seems. A vibration may feel like disaster, but it might just be weeds on the prop. Always check the simple stuff first.

The most important lessons rarely come with applause. They come with silence, tears, and a quiet kind of strength.

There is no autopilot for marriage. Like the boat, it demands constant attention, manual correction, and mutual grace.

Even the worst days have something to teach. If you let them, they will shape you into someone steadier, humbler, and more prepared for what comes next.

CHAPTER 09
ROCKS AND REVELATION

March 20- The sun was dropping fast, painting the lagoon in molten gold and deep gray. The wind from the Atlantic whipped across the shallows as I scanned the depth finder—and held my breath.

That evening marked the end of one of our longest cruises—101 miles from Fort Pierce to Mosquito Lagoon—and I struggled to unwind after a long day of dodging marine traffic and threading through tricky waters.

I circled the anchorage, checking for enough depth to swing safely overnight.

Anchoring can trigger anxiety in even the most seasoned boater. There are so many potential points of failure.

Did the anchor set? Will it hold when the boat swings? Will a tide shift leave me aground? Are there nearby boats I might hit if we drag?

You spend the night half-asleep, listening for anchor alarms and watching the anchor lights of the boats around you—hoping they stay exactly where they're supposed to.

I finally selected a spot and dropped the anchor. It bit like a rabid dog.

I should've felt relief. I didn't.

I spent the night worried I'd snagged a log and wouldn't be able to get the anchor up the next morning.

Looking back, it was foolish to let success turn into fear—but that's what anxiety does. It steals joy and isn't easily done with you.

And it wasn't done with me yet.

Anxiety affects me like a quiet storm—one that brews below the surface, even when everything on the outside seems calm. It doesn't always roar in with panic. More often, it creeps in subtly, like background static I can't turn off.

It speeds up my thoughts, makes small problems feel enormous, and convinces me that if I don't control every detail, everything will fall apart.

It shows up as restlessness when I'm trying to relax. As tension in my shoulders when nothing is visibly wrong. As the constant rehearsal of *what if* scenarios, most of which never happen.

It robs me of presence—pulling me out of the moment and into imagined futures I can't control.

When anxiety is at its worst, even success feels suspicious.

I'll drop anchor safely, then lie awake all night wondering what I did wrong. I'll navigate a difficult stretch, then fixate on the next challenge instead of celebrating what we just accomplished.

It's exhausting. Not loud, not dramatic—but constant. And it shapes the lens through which I see the world, narrowing my focus until all I can spot are the risks.

But naming it—calling it what it is—has helped. Anxiety isn't the truth; it's just a filter. And on the Loop, slowly, I started learning how to see beyond it.

That night in Mosquito Lagoon was just the beginning.

I was starting to realize how often anxiety hijacked my ability to enjoy the moment. Even when everything went right, my mind still braced for what might go wrong.

I chalked it up to inexperience at first, but the pattern kept repeating—and I began to see it for what it really was.

The deeper we got into the Loop, the more clearly I understood: anxiety wasn't just a passing emotion; it was something living under the surface, waiting to surface again—especially in the most beautiful, but demanding, parts of the journey.

And nowhere did that quiet storm rage louder than in the most visually stunning—and perilous—waters we encountered.

The Rocks of Canada

There's nothing quite as intimidating as the Canadian leg of the Loop. While its beauty is undeniable—breathtaking landscapes, pristine waters, and wild serenity—it comes with a constant sense of danger.

From July 19 to August 27, we navigated 713 miles of some of the most jaw-dropping scenery we'd ever seen... and some of the most nerve-wracking. Why? Rocks.

Rocks on the shoreline. Rocks jutting just above the surface. Rocks lurking silently just beneath the waterline. Rocks everywhere—immovable hazards waiting to shear off a prop or punch a hole in your hull.

Boats sink in the Georgian Bay and North Channel for one reason: they hit rocks. And that reality demands constant vigilance. Every day. Every mile. Every moment.

Our boat was no stranger to the Loop. She'd completed it twice before—most recently in 2023 under the command of Mike H. But even a seasoned vessel with a capable captain isn't immune to the risks.

Somewhere just shy of Big Sound, Ontario, heading into an anchorage, Mike H. struck a rock hard enough to land *PATIENCE* (then known as *GRACEFUL WATERBUG*) on the hard for three weeks at Wright's Marina on Parry's Island.

That story haunted me as we crept through those waters, fully aware of what could happen.

It was in the midst of all that beauty—completely mesmerized by the natural splendor—that my anxiety surged to the surface.

The tension between awe and fear was overwhelming, a daily tug-of-war between wonder and caution.

Before this trip, I didn't even realize I struggled with anxiety. Jo-anne—who's dealt with it for years—was the one who helped me recognize the signs in myself. She gently pointed out what I was experiencing and helped me realize I'd been living with anxiety all along.

She's still teaching me how to manage it, and that understanding has made a huge difference—both on the water and now, back on land.

My efforts to manage the anxiety—both the emotional kind and the rocky kind—didn't come soon enough for me to fully enjoy Canada.

We skipped several stunning anchorages simply because I wasn't willing to take the risk. In hindsight, my anxiety robbed me of some truly remarkable moments.

But that's exactly how anxiety works, isn't it? It convinces you to play it safe, to pull back, to say no. And in doing so, it quietly steals the very moments you set out to find.

I've always been driven by goals, and the Great Loop was no exception. What started as an adventure slowly shifted into a quest. Somewhere along the way, the finish line became the focus.

I set my sights on earning that gold AGLCA burgee—granted only to those who complete the Loop—and I zeroed in on it like a man chasing a prize.

It wasn't a new pattern for me. My mind has always lived miles down the road, rarely content to sit in the moment. That trait helped me in business, but out on the water, it began to work against me.

The Moment I Missed

We had planned to break the trip up with a few visits home. One of those centered around a major life event—the birth of our sixth grandchild, a beautiful little girl named Charlee. She was born while we were somewhere near the top of the Georgian Bay in Canada.

Joanne and I had been present for the birth of all five of our previous grandchildren. Missing this one broke our hearts.

A few weeks later, when we cleared customs and re-entered the U.S. at Drummond Island, Joanne flew home to meet Charlee.

I stayed behind.

I told myself the boat needed me. That we were in unfamiliar waters. That I couldn't risk leaving things unattended.

But the truth—when I finally forced myself to face it—was simpler and harder.

I was afraid.

Afraid that if I stepped off the boat, I might not get back on. Afraid that if I paused the journey, I'd lose momentum. I'd worked so hard to get this far—thousands of miles from home—and the job wasn't done. The goal hadn't been reached.

So I stayed.

And I delayed meeting my newborn granddaughter.

Charlee, if someday you read this, please know: it wasn't the Loop that kept me from you. It was anxiety. And I regret that more than I can say.

Now, with the Loop behind me, I see how deeply anxiety shaped that choice. I'm working to rewrite that part of me. These days, I'm learning to recognize fear dressed up as responsibility, and I'm doing the hard work of setting new priorities.

I won't let anxiety steal from me again—especially not the moments that matter most.

Charting a New Course: My Practices for Calming the Waters

It took the Loop to show me something I'd missed my entire life: I'd been living with anxiety, and I didn't even know it.

I had always called it "intensity" or "drive." I thought I was just wired that way—focused, high-energy, always pushing toward the next thing.

But it wasn't just zeal. It was anxiety.

And over time, it had shaped how I related to the world, how I led, how I loved, and how I handled uncertainty.

Being on the water stripped everything down. It exposed the undercurrents I'd learned to ignore.

I began to see myself more clearly—not just intense, but controlled by fear of what might happen and an obsession with making sure things went the way I wanted.

That's not passion. That's pressure. And it was silently eating me alive.

With Joanne's help, and a lot of soul-searching, I began learning how to deal with anxiety in new ways. These weren't instant fixes, but rather daily habits—small shifts in mindset and behavior that started to calm the waters, inside and out.

Here are a few things that helped me most:

Mental Anchors

Name it. When I started saying, "This is anxiety," something shifted. Awareness alone took away some of its power.

Mindfulness. I began practicing deep breathing—just simple 5-5-5 breathing: inhale for 5, hold for 5, exhale for 5. Slowing down helped clear the mental clutter.

Challenge the voice in your head. I asked myself, "Is this fear based in reality? Is it helping me?" Most of the time, the answer was no.

Visual recall. I'd picture a calm anchorage or the stillness of a sunrise over the water. It helped me reset, even in chaotic moments.

Physical Habits

Move daily. Whether it was walking the docks, stretching on deck, or climbing down to the engine room, physical movement helped burn off nervous energy.

Cut back on caffeine and sugar. Both had a way of cranking up my nerves without me noticing—until I did.

Eat to stay steady. I learned to fuel myself with more care—protein, whole foods, fewer simple carbs. It helped more than I expected.

Life Rhythms That Made Space

Build margin. I learned the hard way that overcommitting myself was a recipe for stress. I needed room to breathe.

Simplify decisions. The more I could automate or pre-decide (meals, routines, bills), the less mental wear and tear I experienced.

Get outside. Just being in nature—on the water, in the woods, or sitting on a porch—helped bring perspective back.

Relational and Spiritual Anchors

Talk to someone. Joanne became my sounding board. Sometimes just saying something out loud is enough to soften its grip.

Pray. Anxiety often flows from a deep need for control. Prayer reminded me I wasn't the one holding the world together.

Serve others. Reaching out to help someone else pulled me out of my own head and gave me back a sense of purpose.

Anxiety didn't vanish, but for the first time in my life, I wasn't being ruled by it. I was learning to steer through it—with more grace, more self-awareness, and far less fear.

That inner journey didn't end when we left the water; it's still unfolding, even here on land.

If you've spent your life charging ahead, always in motion, rarely stopping to ask *why you're so tense, so driven, or so worn out*—I'd encourage you to pause. Ask the hard questions. You might discover, like I did, that there's more going on beneath the surface than you realized.

Admitting you're anxious isn't a sign of weakness—it's a step toward freedom. It's saying, *This isn't how I want to live anymore,* and *I'm ready to find a better way.*

And slowly, it's working. The changes I've made—mentally, emotionally, physically—are beginning to bear real fruit. I've even been able to cut back my blood pressure meds, and there's a chance I'll come off them completely.

It might be an overstatement to say the Loop saved my life... but then again, maybe it's not.

What I do know is this: it helped me see the rocks beneath the surface—the hidden hazards I'd been sailing over for years without noticing.

And it offered revelation, too. Not in loud, dramatic flashes, but in quiet moments of clarity—when fear gave way to presence, and I learned, finally, to navigate by something deeper than anxiety.

LOOP LESSONS FROM "BETWEEN ROCKS AND REVELATION"

Anxiety is a thief. It doesn't always roar in—it sneaks in quietly and steals joy from even the most beautiful moments.

Success doesn't silence anxiety. You can do everything right and still lie awake wondering what went wrong. Naming that pattern is the first step to changing it.

Beautiful places don't eliminate fear—they expose it. The stunning waters of Canada revealed just how deeply anxiety lived in me.

Fear dressed as responsibility is still fear. Skipping Charlee's birth wasn't duty—it was avoidance. Facing that truth has helped reshape my priorities.

Don't mistake drive for health. What I called intensity was often unmanaged anxiety. The Loop stripped away the noise and helped me see the difference.

Missing moments leaves a mark. Some regrets—like not meeting my granddaughter—become turning points if you let them.

Growth starts with awareness. Joanne helped me see what I couldn't: that anxiety had shaped much of my life. Recognizing it was a breakthrough.

Discomfort brings clarity. Revelation didn't come despite the anxiety; it came *through* it, like light cutting through fog.

Stillness is strength. Moments of calm—on the water, in prayer, in nature—became anchors that steadied me when storms rose inside.

You can't avoid the rocks, but you can learn to navigate them. What once felt like a threat became a teacher. And I'm still learning.

CHAPTER 10
THE LONG GOODBYE, THE QUIET HELLO

October 11-- That was the day we pulled into Green Turtle Bay, directly behind our buddy boat, *Soul of a Sailor*. We took turns leading, and today we followed Chad and Nancy for the last time—45 miles from Paducah, Kentucky.

In the early morning hours, the river was cloaked in the heaviest fog I'd ever seen on the water. Visibility was so poor, I couldn't even see their stern, though we were only a few hundred feet behind.

A low hum from our engines drifted through the fog as we ghosted forward, reverent in our silence.

A small pod of five Looper boats crept along in single file. We barely moved until we left the Ohio River and turned onto the Cumberland.

Just like that, the fog lifted—like a curtain rising—and revealed a perfect fall day.

At the end of the Cumberland River stands the Barkley Lock—the gateway to my old stomping grounds: Kentucky Lake and the Tennessee River.

We'd heard rumors of long delays; some Loopers had waited hours to get through. But heaven smiled on us. The doors opened, and we motored right in.

Just thirty minutes later, we were rounding the final bend into Green Turtle Bay. It had taken 7 hours to cover the 45 miles.

It was a bitter-sweet moment—Chad and Nancy were about to cross their wake. Their Loop was complete. They had done it. Our months of traveling together were over.

Joanne captured the moment on our Facebook page—*Soul of a Sailor* easing into the harbor, greeted by a chorus of boat horns and a dock full of smiling faces. There was something timeless about it.

We all tied up and hurried to their slip to join the celebration.

Champagne corks popped. Laughter echoed across the water. And the prized gold AGLCA burgee was proudly mounted on *Soul of a Sailor's* burgee staff. It was joy. It was pride.

And it was the beginning of our goodbye.

That night, we gathered at the Tiki Turtle for dinner and live music. The marina glowed behind us in the soft October twilight. I cherish the photos from that evening. I always will.

Our friendship will live on—we still see Chad and Nancy post-Loop—but it's different now. The Loop bonded us like family. We had traveled over 2,900 miles of water together.

As we soaked in the emotion of that day, another familiar face appeared at the docks. Our first real Looper friends—Mark and Terry aboard *Annie Marie*—were here too. We hadn't seen them since July on the Erie Canal, back in Brewerton, New York.

They'd gotten ahead of us and ended up stuck here waiting on parts. It was an unexpected reunion—but one that felt written into the script.

The Next Chapter

We stayed at Green Turtle Bay for a week, blending celebration with a bit of necessary maintenance.

Did I mention I hit a log on the way into Angelo Towhead anchorage—where the Mississippi meets the Ohio River, 134 miles upstream? I did.

It bent a prop just enough to require a haul-out and a prop tuning. Nothing a couple thousand dollars couldn't fix. *Ha.*

While we were still at Green Turtle, we heard our first "Mayday" call—a chilling milestone.

A Looper couple had left the marina earlier that afternoon, planning to anchor several miles south. As they eased into the anchorage, they struck something hard enough to tear the shaft from their boat. Water poured in fast. They feared they'd sink.

Thankfully, they were close enough for help to reach them in time. A service boat arrived quickly, plugged the breach, and towed them back to safety.

It was a sobering reminder: we're all just one decision—or one moment—away from our own "Mayday" call.

With the celebrations winding down and *PATIENCE* back in shape, our time at Green Turtle Bay was drawing to a close. Our eyes began to turn south, toward home.

It surprised me when I caught myself feeling eager to move on. I knew we'd be alone for this stretch, but I felt strangely ready.

Our time at Green Turtle had begun to feel heavy, and I sensed it was time to keep moving.

Leaving friends behind was painful—but the pull of discovery was stronger than the comfort of familiarity.

And I liked that feeling. It felt like growth. Like adventure. Like confirmation that my soul was on the right path.

"This is what feeling alive is like," I told myself. It was real, present, and deeply motivating.

In that moment, I felt it in my bones—it was time to finish what we started.

Farewell To Friends

The day began with the sad business of leaving. We pointed *PATIENCE* south for the final stretch of our journey—from Green Turtle Bay Marina in Grand Rivers, Kentucky, down to the finish line in Destin, Florida.

Chad and Nancy's wake-crossing celebration was behind us. We said our goodbyes—to them, to Mark and Terry, to Annie the pup, and to the many Loopers who had filled our days with laughter, guidance, and companionship.

With farewells complete, it was time to go.

I fired up the engines and moved through my checks with a quiet confidence—one forged through repetition and experience. Normally, I'd let the engines warm for ten minutes or so, but today I lingered. I was stalling, and I knew it.

This moment carried weight.

It was the first time since July that we were pulling away from a marina alone.

The last solo departure had been back in Oswego, New York, when we crossed Lake Ontario and reconnected with *Soul of a Sailor* for a wonderful two month adventure in Canadian waters.

This time was different.

Something about those final 862 miles felt like they were meant for just the two of us. It would be a quieter stretch—one filled with reflection, peace, and a sense of confidence.

We needed that space—not just to finish the Loop, but to absorb what it had truly meant. To reflect. To let it settle in our bones.

There were other loops quietly closing, too—chapters in our lives that had run their course. It was time to release what had been familiar and make room for whatever came next.

As I now reflect on it, I see that the Loop was, in many ways, an exercise in letting go.

With every mile we cruised, another shackle slipped off—almost without notice. I didn't fully grasp it while it was happening. Only later did I understand what had been gradually stripped away.

The Loop brought me back to baseline. It peeled off layers I didn't even know I was wearing. It exposed who I was beneath the busyness, the expectations, the noise—who I was at my core.

The longer we traveled, the more the guilt faded—the guilt of unplugging, of stepping away from obligations, roles, and rhythms I thought I couldn't live without. Somewhere along the way, it felt like I held a quiet funeral for all of that.

And like any loss, there was a kind of mourning. Not sadness, really—but something more like cleansing. A deep, necessary purging.

I'll be honest—I didn't plan for any of this. Some Loopers keep it surface-level. We could've made it just a long boat ride by staying emotionally detached.

But if I had done that—if I had kept it shallow—I would have missed the real treasure. The Loop wasn't just a journey of miles; it was a journey of the soul.

By letting go of the familiar, I made room for something quieter, deeper, more lasting. I wasn't just heading south—I was heading inward, toward a version of myself I might never have met any other way.

From Following to Leading

There was a sense of purpose in taking this final leg alone—just the two of us.

This last leg would be different. Yes, we cruised alongside boats like *Valkyrie, Back Forty,* and *Hawkins Landing* from time to time—but something had shifted.

We met new Loopers who now looked to *us* for guidance. They asked questions. They wanted advice. They saw us as seasoned.

And maybe... they were right.

At first, I didn't accept it. I still felt like a novice. But somewhere along the way, I had crossed my own threshold.

I did know what I was doing.

The Loop had seasoned me. Chad and others had helped shape me. They taught me, encouraged me, and passed on their wisdom.

Now, it was my turn to give back.

That's one of the most beautiful parts of the Great Loop—there's always someone ahead of you helping you grow, and someone behind you waiting for a hand.

Maybe this final stretch wasn't just chance. Maybe it was divine design—a solo run to the finish line, meant to test and transform us one last time.

And it did.

It proved to be the most life-changing leg of the entire journey.

As I write this chapter, I find myself scrolling through old photos and journal entries— hoping to reconnect with the final stretch of the journey home. It doesn't take long.

The memories rush in like a summer squall, and suddenly, I'm there again.

I can feel the gentle sway of *PATIENCE* beneath my feet, the scent of river water in the air, and the soft brush of wind on my face.

That memory opened the door to so many more—each one anchored in a place, a feeling, a stretch of water that marked the journey home.

Panther Creek

We had originally planned to reach Paris Landing that first day, but just shy of the marina, we spotted a quiet anchorage at Panther Creek and decided to pivot. I'm so glad we did.

That evening, we took the dinghy to shore and wandered a wooded trail in perfect solitude.

The water was still, the fall air crisp, and the world felt beautifully distant. It was as if the Loop had gifted us a sacred pause to recalibrate and recover from the fresh emotions of leaving our friends, and the changes it brought.

We didn't say much during those first few hours underway, but that night, as the sun set and we sat together on the bow, the words finally came.

Kenny Chesney played softly in the background, singing, *"Boats... vessels of freedom, harbors of healing."* It was the perfect soundtrack. He gave voice to what we were just beginning to put into words.

As Chesney's music played on, we really did have a *"beautiful view of the end of the world"* from here.

In fact, it felt like I could see *both* ends of the world.

Over my shoulder was the old world—the one I left behind 4,700 miles ago. It had been a good life, full of meaning and milestones.

It shaped me, carried me, and eventually brought me here, to the bow of this boat, on this quiet evening, between tides—one going out, one coming in.

And ahead of me was the new one. A world where I'd reclaimed my-self—my love of life, my sense of adventure, my capacity for growth and peace. In this stillness, I saw how far I'd come—and how much more life there was to live.

As we lingered in the sunset, we unpacked our memories—lessons learned, emotions stirred, moments of growth—and marveled at the peace the water now gave us so freely.

It was a perfect transition.

Back in Destin, when we first cast off, that departure was chaotic and clumsy—shadowed by nerves and uncertainty. But now, with 4,773 miles behind us, everything had changed. The fear was gone. The hesitation had faded.

We knew the boat, and more importantly, we knew ourselves. This water had become more than an adventure. It had become our home. Maybe even our sanctuary.

We felt happily alone that night, in a good way. But the Loop never failed to surprise us. More was on the way.

LOOP LESSONS – THE RIVER CALLED ME HOME

Some goodbyes are beginnings in disguise. Letting go of friends like Chad and Nancy wasn't just an end—it was the opening of a quieter, more personal chapter.

Stillness reveals what motion hides. Slowing down—at Panther Creek or in moments of solitude—allowed space for deeper truths to surface.

The journey inward is just as real as the miles traveled. As we turned south, we weren't just completing a route—we were discovering parts of ourselves we hadn't met before.

Letting go makes space for what matters. Releasing expectations, titles, and busyness was necessary to hear the quieter voice within.

You won't know you've changed until you're tested. In those final miles, we realized how much wisdom and confidence we had quietly earned.

Mentorship is a sacred chain. We were shaped by those ahead of us, and in time, began offering our hand to those coming behind.

The real journey starts when the noise fades. Beyond the celebrations and the checklists, the Loop left us with something more enduring: a deeper understanding of who we are.

Leadership doesn't mean knowing everything—it means showing up with humility and hard-won experience.

Home isn't always a place. Sometimes it's the peace you find when you're exactly where you're meant to be.

The Loop isn't just a journey across water—it's a passage through your own life. Each mile reveals more of who you truly are.

CHAPTER 11
THE RIVER CALLED ME HOME

As I sat down to write this chapter, I gave myself some time to scroll through old photos and notes—hoping to reconnect with the final stretch of the journey home. It didn't take long.

The emotions came rushing in, and suddenly I was back on the Loop. I could almost feel the gentle sway of the boat beneath me, smell the water in the air, and feel the wind brushing across my face.

If these pages end up tear-stained, know this: the tears aren't just salty—they're sweet.

Familiar Waters

After that unforgettable night at Panther Creek, we awoke to the magic of the Tennessee River. A thick morning fog hung low over the water, and as we floated in the stillness, it felt like we were suspended between worlds.

I sipped coffee on the back deck, watching the fog slowly lift like a veil. We had only eight miles to cruise that day—down to Paris, Tennessee—but I had been waiting for this stretch.

These were my waters. My roots.

Of all 6,000 miles of the Loop, this was the only stretch that was familiar. I had spent some of my best teenage years right here.

As the fog gave way to a clear morning sky, we raised anchor and began a four-day run through the waters that had shaped my youth.

We spent the night at Paris Landing, then set out the following morning for Pebble Isle Marina—where an unexpected surprise awaited me.

PIVOT

It's hard to overstate the influence of a mentor—especially one who never knew they held that role.

For us, that mentor was the crew of PIVOT, Elliot, and Jennifer, who inspired us long before we ever left the dock. In fact, Joanne might never have agreed to this journey if it weren't for their YouTube channel, *Scho and Jo*.

A particularly memorable moment came when they released their two-and-a-half-hour documentary, *From Zero to Gold,* chronicling their Great Loop adventure and culminating in their emotional Wake Crossing.

We were cruising through the Chesapeake when it premiered, and there was something electric about watching their story unfold while we were right in the middle of writing our own.

We watched it wide-eyed and grinning, pointing at familiar marinas and anchorages, swapping stories about the places we'd shared.

It stirred something deep in us—a rising anticipation for our own Wake Crossing, and the emotions we knew would come with it.

In short, they fed the dream. They gave it shape. And they gave us the courage to chase it.

It was a powerful reminder that what you allow into your mind is shaping you—whether you realize it or not.

PIVOT had been sold after Elliot and Jennifer completed their Loop to a young couple, Frances and Nils—who later took her back out on the Loop themselves.

On October 21, we pulled into Pebble Isle Marina. Later that afternoon, I noticed a boat approaching the docks that caught my eye.

It was *PIVOT*. She was pulling in right behind us.

I made my way to the dock and positioned myself to catch their lines and welcome them in. I can't quite explain why, but touching those lines—placing my hand on her rail—felt almost magical.

I had followed along for two years as this little boat made its way around the Loop. She had symbolized the dream, taught me, and kept me moving.

And now, there she was—real, tangible, docked right behind us. This wasn't just a YouTube story anymore. It was real life, right in front of me.

Frances and Nils were gracious. They let me gawk a little, and we chatted for a while.

They had no way of knowing what that boat meant to me. For a moment, I felt like I'd met a rock star.

That evening, we all gathered on another Looper boat for docktails and conversation—a night full of laughter, stories, and reflection.

It was one of those moments you don't forget.

Loops Within the Loop

There are many loops that close as you make your way around. Incomplete parts of yourself find completion. Open wounds in your psyche find sutures. Unwritten songs find their tune. Unfinished chapters are written. Past failures are put to bed. Circles are closed.

We were now closing circles we didn't even know were open.

Leaving Chad, Nancy, and the rest of our friends behind at Green Turtle Bay was one loop closing—the loop of shared miles, laughter, and companionship.

Meeting PIVOT closed another loop—the loop of our beginning. The dream that had once only lived on a screen was now tied up at the dock beside us, tangible and real.

In that moment, I was able to say *thank you*—and to recognize something deeper: I no longer needed PIVOT.

I had lived vicariously through her once, but now I was living the dream for myself. Her job was done. The circle was complete.

I couldn't help but wonder what other loops—emotional, spiritual, unseen—were quietly coming full circle as we continued south at ten knots.

One thing was certain: mile by mile, the Loop was offering me a sense of closure—a quiet, deep satisfaction I had been seeking for a long time.

Back to Where It Began

"Oh, Tennessee River and a mountain man, we get together anytime we can."

That line from Alabama's first big hit in 1980—*Tennessee River*—was more than just a catchy chorus. It was in the soundtrack of my life.

I played it often, and for good reason: during those years, I was lucky enough to be working and living on the Tennessee River.

The song wasn't just background music—it mirrored my days, my surroundings, and the life I was building.

Returning to the Tennessee River aboard *PATIENCE* was a homecoming. The scenery hadn't changed much—broad, winding water framed by bluffs and trees—but I had.

This wasn't just another stretch of the Loop; it was something deeper. A loop within the Loop. My life was bending back to its roots, to the place where I first started becoming a man.

As a teenager, the Tennessee River meant everything. It was wild and beautiful and full of opportunity. The outdoors lit me up—gave me purpose and space to grow.

I started college early, just seventeen, but school wasn't the only thing on my mind. I had a plan.

First Steps to Manhood

In April of 1979, I walked into a local bank in Big Sandy, Tennessee, and somehow—God only knows how—convinced them to give me a loan. I used the money to buy an old Chevy truck and some diving gear.

If I had a photo of that truck today, I'd frame it. I wish I still had it. It rattled and roared and never let me down.

The plan was simple: dive for freshwater shells. There was a good market back then—Asian pearl farmers used the mother-of-pearl as seed nuclei. Occasionally, a shell had a pearl of its own, and that brought in extra cash.

It was hard work in murky waters, but it paid off.

I built my own Hookah rig from a gas-powered compressor, a tangle of hoses, and pipe I pieced together. No YouTube. No manual. Just teenage stubbornness and a drive to make it work.

My dad let me convert his John boat into a dive boat, and I was in business.

For two summers, I dove that river—hour after hour, day after day. I could make $300 a day, which in the early '80s felt like striking gold.

I'd come home sun-drenched and bone tired, but I was learning independence and resilience without even knowing it.

When we entered those familiar waters on the Loop, I expected nostalgia. What I didn't expect was how deeply it would hit me.

Here I was again, back where my story of manhood had begun. Those summers weren't just about making money—they were about making me. Every hour underwater, every breath through that homemade rig, was shaping the person I would become.

Where did that young guy go? The one who dove these waters for shells and chased success with nothing but grit and raw ambition?

I know how I see myself now—older, seasoned, and successful by my own measure. But what would he think if he looked at me today? Would he be proud—or disappointed?

I hoped he'd smile. Maybe even nod in quiet approval, recognizing that while the man had changed, the core of him—the hungry, curious, adventurous part—was still alive, even 44 years later. Still chasing something real on the water.

Diving the river was tough work. Visibility back then was nearly zero.

I'd crawl along the bottom with a gunny sack tied around my neck, collecting shells entirely by feel.

I have so many stories from those days—like the time I wriggled under an overturned boat and completely lost my bearings. Or the time I got tangled in an abandoned trot line, hooks snagged all over me. I had to cut myself free, blind in the dark water.

It all came rushing back—the smells, the sounds, the weight of the river.

But more than that, *he* came back. The young man I'd nearly forgotten. The guy with cuts on his hands and big dreams. It was good to see him again in those waves... and to remember his fire.

Each bend in the river brought another memory. Each quiet anchorage reminded me of the boy I'd once been. Something stirred at the helm that day—like time folding in on itself.

There's a strange kind of peace in retracing the water that once carried you forward.

I remembered who I was then—a young guy chasing money and meaning, full of ideas but still forming. And I realized how much had changed.

The Loop wasn't just taking me to new places—it was tethering me to old ones. It reminded me that even as I seek new horizons, I'm shaped by the currents I came from.

I'm not that kid anymore—scraping river mud from my wetsuit or fighting to keep my gear working. Life has moved on. But cruising those familiar waters helped me reconnect with the version of me who first learned to hustle, to fix what was broken, to carve out a life with his own hands.

The Tennessee River was where I first learned to breathe deeply underwater—literally and figuratively.

The Loop brought me back, not just to remember, but to integrate. To carry forward the grit and hope of that young diver and merge it with the man I am today.

The Loop doesn't erase your past. It refines it. It reframes it. It lets you loop back—not to relive who you were, but to honor him... and then keep going.

LOOP LESSONS – A LOOP WITHIN THE LOOP (REFINED VERSION)

Some places carry more than memories—they carry the blueprint of who you once were.

Dreams need fuel, and mentors provide the spark. Following *PIVOT's* journey gave us courage before we ever cast off.

You never know who you're shaping. The example you live may quietly launch someone else's greatest leap.

Closure doesn't always announce itself. Some of the most meaningful loops close in quiet places—anchored in fog, on familiar waters, or beside a dream made real.

The Loop doesn't just move you forward—it folds time, letting past, present, and future meet in the current.

Reconnection is a form of discovery. Sometimes the path ahead only becomes clear when you remember where you started.

The things that once inspired you may someday need to be released. Touching *PIVOT's* rail was both a thank you and a farewell. Her work in my story was complete.

The boy who dove these waters didn't vanish—he matured. And the best gift I could give him was to finish what he started.

The river didn't just carry me home—it carried me back to who I've always been, and forward to who I was becoming.

CHAPTER 12
FAMILY TIDES

By late October, fall was in full swing. The trees lining the riverbanks wore the bronzed glow of a long, hot summer, their leaves now bursting with vibrant color. The air had turned crisp, especially in the early mornings.

As we passed through Pickwick Lock and entered Mississippi, I was stunned by the unexpected beauty of this stretch of the state.

We spent a few days in Counce, Tennessee, at Grand Harbor Marina. We rode our e-bikes through the wooded trails and I fished in the evenings.

From there, we made a side trip up the Tennessee River to Florence. Two special things awaited us.

Muscle Shoals, Alabama.

Sitting just across the river from Florence, Muscle Shoals holds a legendary place in American music history as the seemingly unlikely birthplace of some of the most influential recordings of the 20th century.

I am a wanna-be musician, and this was more than cool to a man who is never too far from a guitar.

Since the 1960s, this small town has been a powerhouse of soul, rock, and R&B. The "Muscle Shoals Sound" was defined in part by a group of local session musicians known as the Swampers, whose deep-groove rhythms and soulful playing attracted the likes of the Rolling Stones, Paul Simon, Bob Dylan, and Lynyrd Skynyrd.

What made Muscle Shoals unique was its unassuming, integrated musical spirit during a time of deep segregation in the South—a place where race didn't matter as much as the music.

It was a treat to see those tiny studios and imagine all the talent that had walked through their doors. And still does.

It was exciting to visit such a historical place. But more exciting things awaited us.

Family Time: Beka's Crew

The biggest reason for our detour to Florence was family.

Our daughter Beka and her crew live only a couple of hours away, and this was the perfect opportunity for a visit. They joined us for the weekend aboard PATIENCE.

It was my first time meeting my newest granddaughter, Charlee—and she captured my heart the moment she smiled at me.

Her sweetness, her calm presence, it all felt like grace. And meeting her out on the water somehow made it even more special. I know I missed her birth, and I carry the weight of that choice—the fear of leaving the boat, the journey, the momentum.

But maybe that's why my heart now ties her to the Loop in such a meaningful way. In a sense, her birth will always be part of this adventure.

With four adults, three kids—including a baby—and limited space, it felt more like a floating campground than a boat. But it was joyful, noisy, and full of laughter.

On Sunday, we took a relaxing day cruise and dropped anchor in a beautiful spot along the river. It was fantastic.

My 14-year-old grandson, Tyler, explored every nook and cranny of the boat, curious about how everything worked.

Tyler spent some time at the helm as we made our way past big barges and followed the winding river. He learned how to read the channel markers and keep us in the safe water. He did great—focused, careful, and curious.

As we talked about how the buoys keep you off the rocks and in the right lane, I found myself smiling at the simple wisdom in it.

"Keep it between the buoys"—it's good advice for boating, but it works pretty well for life too. Stay focused. Pay attention to the signs. Don't drift too far off course. Simple, steady, and solid.

He also discovered a love for fishing. He spent most of his time with a rod in hand, perfectly content to cast lines and watch the water, lost in the quiet rhythm of it all.

The rest of us worked hard to keep the three-year-old, Cowan, safely inside the rails.

It was a special weekend—one of three visits they'd make before our journey ended. We treasured each one.

Family Time: Beth's family on the Erie Canal

Before Florence, though, came another unforgettable family moment—this one way up north.

While we were on the Erie Canal, we were blessed by a visit from our daughter Beth, her husband Heath, and their three kids—Katy, Kamden, and Kenzlee.

It was July, and the northern waters were a cool relief from the summer heat.

Unfortunately, PATIENCE was "in the hospital," so to speak—waiting on engine parts that left us stranded in Brewerton, NY for two weeks.

Our plan had been to cruise the rest of the Erie Canal together, but we were stuck at the dock. Still, we made the most of it.

The kids—ages 11, 9, and 5—loved sleeping onboard. Each night, the salon was transformed into a floating dorm room. Kamden ended up sleeping underneath the table, while the other two shared the pullout bed.

Kamden and Katy loved fishing off the dock and watching the steady parade of boats go by. They peppered us with questions about boat life, curious about how everything worked.

And then there was Kenzlee—wide-eyed and full of energy. I'll never forget that tiny, 25-pound girl, always strapped into a life jacket, darting around the deck like a squirrel hunting for a nut. She brought pure joy to every corner of PATIENCE.

I loved watching the kids explore and learn about the water. I found myself hoping they might grow to love it the way I do.

More than that, I wanted to share the connection I feel out there—the peace, the clarity, the sense of something bigger.

Maybe, just maybe, being on the boat would plant a seed that helps them one day understand what *Blue Mind* is really all about.

A Looper's gift

Just as we were feeling the sting of missing our planned Erie Canal cruise, one of those small miracles the Loop is known for quietly showed up.

Another Looper boat, TREASURE STATE, happened to be docked alongside us. We had first met Alan and Pam back in the Chesapeake, at St. Michaels.

When they saw the disappointment in our grandkids' faces, they did something extraordinary—they offered to take our family on a day cruise across Oneida Lake to Sylvan Beach.

It was a perfect Upstate New York summer day. The kids enjoyed swimming, ice cream, and sunshine. A memory we'll never forget.

Generosity is the norm in the Looper community. People like Alan and Pam showed my family that kindness isn't the exception—it's the culture.

Afterward, we rented a car and explored the region. We visited Alexandria Bay, toured Boldt Castle and Singer Castle, and wandered through charming small towns.

We also crossed into Canada and spent a few days exploring Niagara Falls.

It was one of those classic family adventures—riding the boats to the base of the falls, snapping photos from every angle, and feeling the mist soak through our clothes.

We hit all the tourist hotspots, from the observation towers to the souvenir shops, and ate ourselves silly along the way.

Ice cream, restaurants, snacks—we didn't hold back. It was loud, chaotic, and absolutely wonderful. A memory-making kind of trip.

While we soaked in the scenery, we also found ourselves observing the people—the way they moved, talked, and engaged with the place.

It became clear that the environments we live in are more than just geography. They shape us.

Geography Is the Stage—But People Are the Story.

I've spent a lot of time reflecting on the places we visited as we rounded the Loop—and the people who call those places home.

It struck me how much the environment we choose to live in shapes the way we see the world. Geography isn't just backdrop; it's a lens. A filter through which life is experienced, values are formed, and character is forged.

On the Great Lakes, for example, you learn quickly to respect the power of water. There's a humility that comes from living beside something so vast and changeable—calm one moment, raging the next.

Down in the Keys, nature weaves itself into daily life. The tides, the coral, the hurricanes—they all remind you how fragile and vibrant the world can be.

And in the Chesapeake Bay, you're constantly surrounded by echoes of American history.

The past lingers there, not just in the architecture or museums, but in the spirit of the people—many of whom carry a deep awareness of sacrifice, freedom, and what it cost to build a nation.

I've never been much for quick vacations—the kind where you drop into a place for a few days, snap some photos, and move on. That's never been enough for me. I prefer immersion.

I want to meet the people, listen to their stories, walk their streets, shop at their markets, and let their rhythms shape me. I want to understand how their environment has molded them—and hopefully adopt a sliver of their worldview into my own.

Each stop along the Loop gave me the chance to do that, and in doing so, I became more rounded. More understanding. More human.

But geography is only the stage. People are the actors. And they are what matter most.

At every stop, I was drawn not just to the scenery, but to the people shaped by it—the dockmasters, the waitresses, the fellow boaters, the local storytellers. These encounters became the soul of the journey.

I believe deeply that where you live shapes who you become. The land, the water, the history—they all work quietly on your spirit.

But in the end, it's not the place that defines the meaning of your story. It's the relationships. It's the characters who walk in and out of your script.

That's the beauty of the journey.

So yes, the setting matters. But I don't want to forget the purpose of the play.

The stage may be striking, but it's the storyline—the people—that make it worth watching. And worth living.

A Hard Truth

That brings me full circle back to my family.

I have another hard confession to make.

For the last 14 years, I'd been a distracted Papa. Not absent. Not unloving. Just not fully present. The Loop didn't just help me see that—it helped me *feel* it. Feel the weight of what I'd been missing.

This journey opened my eyes to the fact that while I had been disengaged in many areas of life, this—*my family*—was where it hurt the most.

I wasn't just robbing them of my presence. I was robbing *myself* of the greatest gift God gives a man: the generations that come after him.

Since returning to "dirt life," I've made a change. I'm more engaged. More present. And I'm better for it. Happier. More grounded.

The Loop gave me many gifts—but none more meaningful than this.

In the end, the most enduring parts of the Loop weren't the waterways or marinas—they were the people.

My grandkids learning to fish, my daughters climbing aboard with their families, the laughter echoing across cramped cabins, the kindness of strangers-turned-friends.

These were the true treasures.

The Loop gave me stunning views and quiet mornings, but more importantly, it gave me time—real, uninterrupted time—with the people I love.

It's the relationships that make the story worth telling.

LOOP LESSONS – FAMILY TIDES

Presence is the real gift. Boats, travel, and adventure are incredible, but nothing compares to being truly present with the people you love. The Loop reminded me that what my family needs most isn't perfection—it's attention.

A cramped boat can hold a lot of love. With four adults and three kids squeezed onto PATIENCE—twice—we learned that tight quarters often create the best memories. The laughter, the chaos, the shared meals and late-night chats made the space feel expansive.

Keep it between the buoys. Watching Tyler learn to steer past barges taught us more than just seamanship. "Stay in the channel" became a guiding metaphor—on the water and in life. Pay attention, adjust when needed, and don't drift too far off course.

Slow moments matter. Evenings spent fishing at Grand Harbor, bike rides through wooded trails, and lazy afternoons at anchor reminded me that not every memory has to be epic. The quiet ones often go deepest.

Pass it on. Watching the grandkids fall in love with the water stirred something in me. I hoped they might carry it forward—that they'd discover their own Blue Mind one day, and remember that peace can be found in rhythm, stillness, and salt air.

The people are the real scenery. Every stop along the Loop was scenic, but what made each one unforgettable were the people—family, friends, fellow Loopers, and strangers who left fingerprints on our journey.

Geography shapes the soul. The places we visited weren't just interesting—they were formative. The Keys, the Great Lakes, the Chesapeake—each one carried lessons, culture, and spirit. Where you live slowly shapes who you become.

Don't just visit—immerse. It's easy to rush through new places, but real connection comes when you slow down, listen, and let the world sink in. Immersion creates empathy, perspective, and lasting memories.

It's never too late to re-engage. I spent years distracted—never absent, just not fully present. The Loop gave me the clarity to change that. Reconnection isn't just possible—it's life-changing.

CHAPTER 13
WHEN THE WATER WHISPERS

At some point, every journey worth taking will carry you into deeper waters—places where clarity, meaning, and even faith begin to surface.

This chapter isn't about doctrine or dogma—it's about presence. About paying attention.

Because when you step into something bold—whether it's the Great Loop or any dream that stretches you—you open yourself to something deeper, more enduring, and far bigger than you imagined.

As we cruised the Tennessee River, I knew that something spiritual was unfolding beneath the surface.

I recalled moments when the water spoke more clearly than words ever could. One early Loop experience captured that truth perfectly.

March 9 began with a bad decision—one shaped by a rough night and sheer exhaustion.

We had left Key West the day before and enjoyed a calm, easy 79 mile run up the east coast to an anchorage at Long Key.

By 4 PM, we had the hook down, dinner served, and a gorgeous sunset glowing across the water. Only three other boats shared the anchorage. It felt peaceful... until it wasn't.

Just as the last light faded, our anchor alarm blared—we were dragging. That night turned into a sleepless vigil. I stayed at the helm, eyes glued to the GPS, repositioning the anchor every couple of hours.

Joanne slept below while I stood watch, too tired and inexperienced to fully diagnose the issue. Only later did I realize the anchor had likely fouled—something I couldn't see or understand in the darkness.

When dawn finally broke over the Atlantic, I was beyond relieved. But I was also drained. And in that fog of fatigue, I made one of the worst decisions of the entire Loop.

We'd already completed two successful offshore crossings: a 167-mile Gulf passage and a 105-mile run from Marco Island to Key West. I was starting to feel confident—maybe too confident.

The forecast looked favorable, and the apps showed calm seas. So I decided to bypass the protected Hawk Channel and head offshore into the Atlantic for what I hoped would be another smooth cruise north toward Miami.

Big mistake.

Not long after we got outside, the wind picked up—fast. Before we could make our turn to head north, we found ourselves 5 or 6 miles offshore, in swells that were truly frightening.

The troughs were so deep I nearly lost the horizon at times. With our 19-foot air draft, those waves had to be at least 12 feet.

The boat was getting hammered. It pitched and rolled violently, dishes flew from cabinets, and anything not tied down was crashing to the floor. It was chaos.

Turning around in those conditions was terrifying, but eventually I managed it, pointing us back northwest and letting the seas follow us instead of beating us head-on. Even then, it felt like some waves might overtake us.

Thankfully, as we neared a reef line, the seas began to break up—offering a reprieve.

Looking back, that day was probably the most danger we ever faced on the Loop. And it hammered home a hard-earned truth: Never underestimate the power of water.

You don't have to be religious to feel that something greater is at work in the world. Most people, at one time or another, sense it — that stillness, that stirring, when nature stops you in your tracks and reminds you how small you really are.

That's what this chapter is about: Presence. Awe.

Out on the Loop, that presence felt especially close. Alone with the sea and sky, with no schedule but the tide, I often found myself reflecting on things I couldn't quite explain.

The power of the ocean. The hush of a wind-less dawn. The way the horizon seemed to stretch into something eternal.

I've come to believe that some truths are ancient — and sacred — even if we don't all agree on their source.

For me, that source is God. The water has a way of bringing God near.

Some say God speaks in a still, small voice. I've come to believe that sometimes His voice rides on the water.

Presence in the Wake

Somewhere along the Great Loop — maybe anchored in the Keys or drifting through the quiet reaches of the North Channel — I knew it wasn't just peace I was experiencing. It was presence. Not mine — His.

Fear and faith often met head-on out there. In those moments, Scripture stopped reading like metaphor and started to feel lived. It wasn't just words on a page; it was muscle memory.

The stories weren't ancient anymore. They were unfolding around me in real time. God wasn't only whispering in the stillness. Sometimes, He was shouting through the swells.

One moonlit night at anchor in the Benjamin Islands, the glassy water mirrored a sky full of stars. The boat barely rocked.

I remember thinking, *If the universe is this vast and yet this gentle, it confirms that the One who set it spinning is both powerful and kind.*

It was a thought that lingered as I drifted into sleep. That night didn't just bring peace—it brought perspective.

And in that quiet, the truths I'd long read in Scripture began to feel newly alive, not as distant words but as something present, embodied, and deeply personal.

Scripture Comes Alive at Sea

It's not surprising, really. The Bible is braided with water stories. From the opening line — *"The Spirit of God was hovering over the face of the waters"* — to the final chapter that speaks of a river of life, water flows through the entire narrative of God and humanity.

"As the deer pants for streams of water, so my soul pants for you, my God." (Psalm 42:1) I'd read that verse for years. But miles from shore, I didn't just understand it — I **felt** it. That aching thirst, that longing for something more, pulsed in rhythm with the waves. It wasn't poetry anymore; it was reality.

Jesus once told a Samaritan woman at a well, *"Whoever drinks the water I give them will never thirst."* (John 4:14) On a boat, you bring every need with you. You feel every limitation, especially fresh water. Tanks must be checked, conserved, treated like liquid gold.

Maybe that's why her story struck me harder out there. Jesus wasn't offering convenience; He was offering **sufficiency** — abundance that refuses to run dry.

The more miles we logged, the more those ancient verses surfaced unbidden. A passing squall would remind me of Noah.

A wind-less channel once reminded me of Elijah's encounter with God—not in the wind, the quake, or the fire, but in a gentle whisper that followed.

That's how it often felt out there—like God wasn't shouting over the chaos, but waiting in the calm that came after. Even a dolphin breaking the surface seemed to echo Job's question: *"Who shut up the sea behind doors when it burst forth from the womb?"*

The Book was no longer a distant artifact; it was a soundtrack.

What the Storms Taught Me

Of course, there were stormy days too. Days when the horizon shrank to a wall of slate and nothing but faith kept the throttles steady. I thought of the disciples in the boat, panicking, waking Jesus as the waves crashed: *"Lord, save us! We're going to drown!"* (Matthew 8:25).

And He did — with a word.

That story didn't feel distant anymore. I had lived that fear. I had cried out those same thoughts. And I had known the hush that follows when He speaks.

Most people pray for God to calm the storm — to make the waves stop. But the Loop shaped a different prayer in me. I began asking for a **seaworthy vessel** and the wisdom to navigate whatever lay ahead.

I stopped expecting ease and started seeking endurance.

God isn't in the business of comfort; He's in the business of transformation. He wasn't trying to smooth the waters; He was strengthening me to sail through them.

In the disciples' case, Jesus didn't just calm the storm — He allowed it, and through it revealed something deeper, something they could never have seen in calm water.

I began to see my own journey the same way.

Maybe God didn't merely permit this trip; maybe He **designed** it, winds and waves included, so that I could discover who He really is and who I might become with Him.

The Loop wasn't just a route on a chart; it was a proving ground for my faith. And the lessons didn't stay on the water.

They followed me home. Now, when life stirs up a storm, I don't just brace for impact — I look for the growth it's offering.

Waves That Whisper

One afternoon on the Tennessee River, the water lay flat as polished stone. The only movement came from our wake and the gentle swirl behind the props.

I cut the engines to idle and let the momentum bleed off until we drifted in silence.

Joanne and I sat on the bow, feet dangling over the edge, saying nothing. We didn't need to. The hush spoke louder than any conversation. In that silence I sensed, more than heard, a whisper: *You are seen.*

It was the same whisper I had felt in storms, in moonlit anchorages, in the solitude of early morning coffee on the bridge. It was subtle, but steady. The kind of voice you only hear when everything else goes quiet.

I can't prove it. No instrument will ever log the coordinates of that assurance. But I know what I felt, and I know how deeply it settled me. Sometimes the loudest sermon is preached by still water.

Currents of Connection

A friend once told me that solitude is God's favorite classroom. On the Loop, I learned why.

With no cell signal and nothing but the slap of wavelets against the hull, my internal noise finally quieted.

That's when the deeper questions rose to the surface: Who am I without the titles? What matters when the shore fades from view? Whose voice will I trust when the Garmin chart plotter goes dark?

The answers didn't arrive in thunderclaps. They came gradually, like incoming tide. I realized that the same force carrying my boat forward was drawing my heart homeward — toward trust, toward gratitude, toward love. The sea was both highway and teacher.

Even in its unpredictability, the water offered clarity. Every sunrise at anchor felt like grace.

Every successful docking after a tough day felt like a kind of benediction. Even our near-misses reminded me: You are not alone.

The Map Beneath the Map

Every mariner knows that charts only tell part of the story. Depth changes. Buoys drift. Storms rearrange shoals overnight.

Yet beneath every chart is a hidden, older map: the contours of the earth, the pull of moon on tide, the unseen hand that holds the ocean in place.

Out there, I began to believe that my life has a hidden map as well, drawn by a cartographer who sees farther than I do.

That belief changed the way I read setbacks.

A mechanical failure became a slowdown, not a sentence. A weather delay transformed into a gift of time — space to breathe, to read, to pray.

Even my miscalculations — like venturing offshore that ill-fated March morning — became mid-course corrections on a chart I hadn't known existed.

Maybe it's not about always choosing the right heading. Maybe it's about trusting that even when you drift, grace can reroute you.

Still Waters, Restored Soul

"He leads me beside still waters. He restores my soul." (Psalm 23:2–3) That's not poetic fluff. That's field-tested truth.

I found restoration not in a sanctuary with stained glass, but in sunrises on mirror-smooth bays, in quiet anchorages where the only sermon was silence.

If you ask me where I encountered God most clearly on the Loop, I'll tell you plainly: **on the water.** In the waiting. In the wonder. And in the stillness.

The water made God feel closer—not because He lives out there, but because *out there,* my distractions faded.

The docklines of my life — ambition, obligation, expectation — loosened. And I drifted into awareness.

Not religion. Not performance. Just being... with Him.

Even now, back on land, I carry those still waters inside me. When deadlines loom or headlines roar, I close my eyes and hear the hush of Georgian Bay, the quiet slap of water on the hull, the low hum of an engine idling in the dawn.

And beneath it all, a whisper:

You are seen. You are loved. Steady ahead.

LOOP LESSONS FROM WHEN THE WATER WHISPERS

Seek Presence, Not Perfection Calm seas are nice, but storms reveal character.

Pray for Seaworthiness Ask less for easy conditions, more for a resilient heart.

Let Silence Speak Turn down the volume of life long enough to hear the whisper.

Read the Hidden Map Trust that setbacks can be mid-course corrections.

Carry the Stillness Home You don't have to be on the water to live in its peace.

Some think faith is something practiced in pews and proven by creeds.

The Loop taught me that faith can also be measured in nautical miles, in weathered lines, in the quiet courage to leave the harbor and trust the chart you cannot see.

And every time I remember that open water, I'm reminded that the voice in the swells still speaks — if I'll only slow down long enough to listen.

CHAPTER 14
DOCK LINES AND WEDDING BANDS

Writing about marriage on the Loop feels a bit like docking in high wind—you've got to approach carefully. Here goes:

BOAT FOR SALE

Not long after we crossed our wake, Joanne and I were walking the dock in Destin when we spotted a sleek 2023 yacht tied up nearby. It was the AGLCA flag on the bow that caught my eye—along with the bold **For Sale** sign hanging from the rail.

A young man stepped out of the nearby boat broker's office.

"Want to take a look?" he asked.

"Absolutely," I said.

She was stunning—practically brand new and outfitted with top-of-the-line everything. I turned to the salesman and asked the question everyone eventually asks on a dock like this:

"How much?"

"One million dollars," he said, like he was reading it off a lunch menu.

I nodded slowly, then asked, "What's her story? I see she's got a Looper flag."

Turns out, the wife had agreed to do the Loop—but only if she could pick the boat. She wanted one that checked every box, and this one did. No doubt about it—she had great taste.

They purchased her brand new in Tampa Bay and set out across the Gulf, headed for Destin to spend a few weeks with family before beginning the official counter-clockwise route.

That was as far as they got.

The Gulf turned rough without warning. When they finally tied up in Destin, she stepped off the boat, looked her husband in the eye, and said, "I'm done. Sell the boat—or do it without me."

End of dream.

As we walked away, I couldn't help but feel grateful we'd already crossed our wake before hearing that story.

If Joanne had heard it when we first came to Destin to tour *PATIENCE*, there's a decent chance she'd have marched straight back to Texas, ordered Tex-Mex, and pretended the whole Loop idea was just another weird dream I had.

But that moment—visualizing that woman stepping off the boat, declaring she was done---highlighted an honest reality: people often have very different expectations of the Loop.

And once you're out there, those inequalities don't stay hidden for long.

Boating Newlyweds

Rarely does a couple begin the Loop on equal footing—one person is often more excited, more confident, or more prepared than the other. That imbalance doesn't stay hidden for long.

And the sea doesn't care how long you've been married or how well you think you know each other. It will test the foundations of your relationship.

Back in our land-based life, we'd developed a rhythm—a comfortable balance. We knew how to navigate each other's quirks and preferences, dividing responsibilities in ways that played to our strengths while respecting each other's space and individuality.

But once we stepped onto the boat, all of that had to be rebuilt. The old rhythms didn't always fit the new reality.

Suddenly, we weren't just managing familiar tasks—we were navigating new fears, shifting roles, and unspoken expectations in a completely foreign environment.

It wasn't just about staying in our lanes. It was about rediscovering each other under a different kind of pressure.

It meant learning how to communicate when the wind was up and tempers were frayed. It meant extending grace when mistakes were made, and finding new ways to be teammates when the rulebook we'd relied on for years no longer applied.

In many ways, it felt like we had just gotten married all over again—only this time, without the honeymoon suite or any realistic expectations.

With marriage, I'd at least watched my parents and had some idea of what to expect. But this? Other than a few YouTube couples—who can easily edit out the messy parts—I had no model for how to balance man, woman, and water.

Learning to be partners out here required new perspective, renewed grace, and the courage to unpack some things we'd kept tucked away for years.

Marriage at Sea Level

We married in 1982—she was 18, I was 20. Some folks said we were too young, but I'd put our 43-year marriage up against the best of them.

For us, marrying young turned out to be a blessing. We didn't just build a life together—we grew up together. Our understanding of each other runs deep; honestly, I can barely remember what life was like before marriage.

We balance each other well.

So, when we set out on the Loop, I figured that dynamic would transfer smoothly to boat life. Me, the Captain. Her, the First Mate. It felt like we were just formalizing the roles we'd always played.

And in some ways, we were.

But as we quickly learned—those titles came with new demands.

Our marriage was already strong when we set out on the Loop. We'd always worked side by side—most of my career was spent working from home, and she was right there with me, stepping in where I fell short, shoring up the gaps.

But this journey stretched us in new ways.

We discovered an entirely different level of "working together." Yes, we were still a team—but this wasn't the familiar kind of teamwork. Cruising the Loop demanded more. It required a deeper connection, an unspoken rhythm.

Out here, success meant becoming intuitive with my First Mate—anticipating each other's moves, staying in sync. We had to move as one—same pace, same cadence—or it wouldn't work.

Back in Time

A year earlier, we had no idea just how much our marriage would be challenged—and changed.

I stood at the helm of our newly purchased 40-foot yacht, gripping the wheel with a confidence I hadn't yet earned, staring out at the Gulf of Mexico.

It stretched before me like an unpredictable business partner—capable of calm collaboration or sudden betrayal.

Just three weeks earlier, I'd been in a swivel chair, not a captain's chair—reviewing contracts, not tide charts.

Now it was 5 a.m. on February 9, and we were easing away from Dog Island under cover of darkness, bound for a full Gulf crossing. The stress hung in the air like fog—thick, heavy, inescapable.

"You sure about this?" Jo called from below, her blonde hair whipping across her face as she stepped onto the upper deck.

"Pretty sure," I said, squinting at the Navionics route. "Just trying to follow the GPS until we clear the inlet—and if all goes well, we'll hit Tarpon Springs by dinner."

She gave me that look—the one that had seen me through a dozen entrepreneurial ventures. The one that said, *I trust you.*

But that steady tone between us wouldn't always hold.

In hindsight, the navigation wasn't the hardest part. Learning how to communicate was.

We were both out of our element, learning as we went, doing our best to survive another day.

The Gulf crossing was one of the riskiest segments of the entire Loop—but for us, it was smooth and uneventful. Pleasant, even.

You might call it the calm before the storm. The Gulf sent a false message that morning: *This might just be an easy trip.*

That crossing felt easy. But in those early days, most things weren't.

That day on the Gulf went smoothly. But back near shore, things like docking—less dramatic, more frequent—became the real tests.

Staying married while docking

If you ask most Loopers, they'll tell you—docking is the most stressful daily chore.

PATIENCE stood 19 feet out of the water, with a fully enclosed upper helm. In heavy wind, she catches air like a sailboat. There's a lot of windage to manage. Many Looper boats are like that. It further complicates the task of docking.

Add to that the reality that marinas are packed with million-dollar boats, tight fairways, and the occasional shared slip with no piling between them, and you've got all the ingredients for a full-blown circus.

We watched more than a few couples along the route yelling, cursing, and chaotically muscling their boats into slips—including ourselves.

It might've been funny if it hadn't hit so close to home.

More than once, I spotted t-shirts and coffee mugs that read, *"I'm sorry for what I said while we were docking."*

Clearly, we weren't alone. Docking has a way of testing not just your seamanship, but your relationship.

It doesn't take long before you start seeking out every tip, trick, and bit of training you can find—anything to make the next approach go smoother.

The gift that saves marriages

When we purchased PATIENCE from Mike and Grayce, they gifted us headsets. It likely saved our Loop.

With them, I didn't have to raise my voice to talk to her. Nobody else had to hear when she scolded me.

And let's be honest, with all the engine noise and other sounds, along with the fact that I was at the helm, with so many blind spots from the bridge enclosure, it was necessary.

Want to save your marriage at the dock? Buy headsets.

Fort Pierce

By the time we pulled into Fort Pierce, Florida, we'd logged around 25 docking experiences. But I knew this one would be different.

Before I get into it, there's a popular saying among Loopers: *"You either watch the show—or you are the show."*

Fort Pierce Marina sits right on the Intracoastal, not far from the inlet, and the currents there are no joke.

We arrived near slack tide, but by the time we fueled up and checked in, the incoming tide was rolling hard.

There was nothing to do but commit. I'd need Joanne's full communication powers, and I'd have to bring my A-game.

We rounded the corner, entered a wide fairway, and I spun PATIENCE to port, using the current to ease us into place.

That's when I noticed the crowd. No exaggeration—at least 15 people were watching from nearby boats, sitting on bows and sterns like they were waiting for a fireworks show.

The guy on the next boat over was on his swim deck, holding a fender in one hand and a boat pole in the other.

Apparently, they'd either heard we were coming—or they'd seen one too many docking disasters lately.

Here's where Joanne really shined. Calm and clear, she called out commands: "A little to starboard. Neutral. Let her drift. Good—now back. Okay, port. Straighten up. Fifteen feet. Starboard again. Five feet. Perfect. Stop."

It was textbook—and all her.

The deckhand caught the lines as Jo tossed them. Not a bump. No pole, no fender needed.

The guy next to us clapped and shouted, "Nice job!"

I gave a casual wave like it was no big deal. But truthfully, my heart was racing and my palms were soaked. I thought, *That might be the best I'll ever do. Maybe we should sell the boat now and go out on a high note.*

The spectators melted away—some relieved, others disappointed the show never materialized.

That Fort Pierce docking showed us what we were capable of—when we truly worked as a team.

But getting there didn't happen overnight. That kind of teamwork had to be learned—and earned—one docking, one misstep, one sharp word at a time.

Expectations

Another thing became obvious early on: I had a problem with expectations.

In my head, it was clear what Joanne *should* be doing when we were docking, locking, or maneuvering. But Jo came into this with zero boating experience. Every task she took on—every line, every lock, every movement—she had to learn from scratch.

She also had to figure out how to communicate under pressure—quickly and clearly—about where the boat was relative to docks, pilings, or other obstacles.

"Left" or "right" didn't cut it. I needed "port," "starboard," "bow," and "stern." And vague terms like "close" or "far" weren't useful—I needed feet, not feelings.

Maneuvering a nearly 45-foot boat is like backing a semi down an icy slope.

There were tears. My words weren't always kind.

I see now that my sharpness came from my own insecurity. When I barked at Joanne about a line or a delay, it wasn't really about her—it was my fear, my frustration, my inexperience boiling over.

And for every mistake she made, I made five.

As the miles passed, I began to see the pattern. When I was overwhelmed, I turned my stress on her. It wasn't fair. And I'm still working to change that.

Somehow, through it all, we kept moving forward—together.

Just PATIENCE—and a little more grace between us than the day before.

We quickly developed a habit: a pre-departure walkthrough where we circled the boat together, talking through every detail. Which line would come off first, how I planned to maneuver, where Joanne needed to be—step by step, we made a plan.

Clear, consistent communication became our anchor—especially when the pressure was on.

We were learning how to read each other better, respond with more grace, and defuse stress before it took over.

By the time we slid PATIENCE into the slip at Destin Harbor Marina and placed the gold burgee on the bow, we had grown. The miles, the missteps, and the countless dockings had shaped us into something stronger—more in sync, more resilient.

We could almost read each other's minds.

The Loop had dismantled our old ways of communicating and rebuilt them into something deeper, more intuitive. It stretched us, refined us, and ultimately brought us closer.

Our marriage is stronger because of it.

If your relationship is strong, it will likely grow stronger. If it's strained, the stress will surface quickly. The Loop doesn't lie—it refines, reveals, and, if you let it, rebuilds.

But if you're willing to grow together, it can turn a good team into a great one.

LOOP LESSONS – DOCK LINES AND WEDDING BANDS

The Loop will test your teamwork—and reveal the cracks. Marriage on land and marriage at sea are not the same. The Loop strips away distractions and demands a new level of partnership, communication, and grace.

Clear communication isn't optional—it's everything. Step-by-step planning, calm language, and shared expectations make the difference between chaos and confidence, especially when docking.

Buy the headsets. Trust us. They don't just improve communication—they protect your dignity, your sanity, and your relationship.

Docking is a mirror. Few things expose your stress patterns like trying to control 20,000 pounds of fiberglass in front of an audience. What shows up at the dock is often what's been simmering beneath the surface.

Strong teams aren't born—they're built, one slip at a time. We didn't become great boat partners overnight. It took repetition, failure, patience, and practice. But by the end, we could move as one.

CHAPTER 15
HAPPY RE-BIRTHDAY TO ME

Happy Re-Birthday to Me: A celebration of change, gratitude, and the woman who made it all possible

It's not hard to explain why my 63rd birthday was so emotional. Sure, I was only 277 miles from achieving a long-standing goal.

But the deeper reasons were more personal—woven into everything this book has tried to capture.

My 62nd year felt like a victory lap—a celebration of what was, and a leaning into what could still be.

It was a spiritual journey, one in which I was cleansed by salt and solitude, reconstituted by wind and water, distilled by miles.

It became a celebration of life, shaped by the experiences and lessons along the way.

I learned patience in the doldrums, courage in the squalls, humility in the currents. I learned to read the sky, trust my instruments, and listen to my instincts.

I discovered the limits of my control—and the depth of my resilience.

All of it—every mile, every lesson—culminated in the most meaningful birthday I've ever had.

A Happy Birthday

The morning of November 6—the day I turned sixty-three—we untied the lines at Bobby's Fish Camp, a rustic, legendary stop along the Great Loop.

It was one of those places every Looper knows, tucked against the riverbank with stories as thick as the fried catfish they used to serve.

Unfortunately, the restaurant closed during COVID, but they still offer Loopers fuel and dockage.

Today was my day, and I got to spend it doing what I loved--at the helm of PATIENCE.

Just a few miles downriver, we approached the Coffeeville Lock—the 123rd and final lock of our Great Loop journey. A quiet milestone, but a profound one.

This was the last gate between us and our return to the sea. From here, the river would run free all the way to the Gulf.

The water was still fresh, but it wouldn't be for long. As it wound southward, it would slowly turn brackish, mingling with the tides of Mobile Bay—just like us, merging something old with something new.

Before writing this chapter I rewatched the video we took as we entered the lock.

The sound of my voice, the ease in my posture—I was light, unguarded, fully present. No strain in my words, no tension in my movements. Just joy. Quiet, unmistakable joy. I was free.

On screen, I watched as we maneuvered the boat with quiet confidence—Jo handling the lines with practiced ease, me at the helm with calm assurance. We moved like a team that had found its rhythm.

I couldn't see it then, not fully—but I recognize it now. We were seasoned. Skilled. At ease. We had become the kind of boaters we used to admire at the start of the Loop.

So different from the wide-eyed rookies who nervously fumbled their way through their first locks months ago.

Last Anchorage

That night we anchored for the last time, on the Tensaw River, beneath a sky that looked painted by God Himself—a watercolor wash that faded from gold to indigo.

Birthdays have never meant much to me—not even as a kid.

I thought back to celebrations from years past: flickering candles in crowded restaurants, gifts I didn't need, laughter that didn't quite reach the soul.

As I've grown older, birthdays have sometimes felt more like quiet reminders of time slipping by—less celebration, more reckoning. Almost painful.

A tally of missed opportunities. A slow dimming of dreams that once burned bright.

But that night on the Tensaw felt different.

There was no regret. No unneeded gifts. No ache for something more. Just Jo, the water, and a quiet certainty that I had finally come home to myself.

The greatest birthday gift I've ever received.

I made a video before dinner, standing alone on the bow as the setting sun turned the sky to cotton candy. My voice caught something true:

"If I had known, as a kid, that 63 would be spent on my own boat, anchored in a place like this..." I said as I gestured over my shoulder. "I would have been all about it. Bring it on. Finish it out with a bang. Let life become what it can be."

The satisfaction on my face is unmistakable.

Watching that clip now brings it all rushing back.

I could feel the freshness of the river air, the hush of evening settling in, the gentle current slipping past the hull.

My hand traced the rail of PATIENCE, grounding me in the moment. Somewhere nearby, a heron called into the dusk.

It was the first birthday in years that felt like a true celebration—and not because of the number. Because of the meaning. And man, did it feel perfect. It felt like magic.

Later, Jo and I sat together on the bow, the water hushed beneath us, the sky painted in fading pastels.

Some views are impossible to put into words—you just have to be there.

That's how I felt looking out at the horizon that night, where the last light of day melted into the stillness of the water.

For once, I wasn't chasing anything. I was exactly where I wanted to be.

Joanne's Gift to me

And when I looked at Joanne, I felt the same way.

No words could capture what I saw—the depth of our shared history, the steady resolve in her eyes, the grace that had carried us through every mile.

Like the water itself, she carried a calm beneath the surface and a beauty that revealed itself in layers.

Sitting beside her in the golden hush of that evening, I wanted to tell her—this was just the close of one chapter in a love story still being written.

I spoke with a new understanding of myself—shaped by the miles behind us, the trials we weathered, and the quiet triumphs that marked our journey.

As we looked out over the stillness, I found myself reflecting on the life we had built together.

We had weathered storms, both literal and emotional, and learned how to trust each other more deeply, to move as a team, to speak with grace and listen with intention.

I told her how grateful I was. Not just for the trip, but for her—her steadiness, her courage, her belief in us. For saying yes to something so uncertain. For making it beautiful.

In that moment, the bow wasn't just the front of the boat—it was a sacred space, a quiet altar where gratitude met memory.

And the woman beside me wasn't just my wife—she was my co-captain, my safe harbor, the truest part of home I'd ever known.

I wanted her to know what a gift she had given me—by being here, by saying yes to this wild, beautiful adventure.

We're very different, she and I. My stubborn drive meets her gracious heart. My intensity is steadied by her calm presence. My headlong passion is grounded by her quiet strength.

She is my refuge, my anchor, the one I dream with and fight for. The only one I ever want to come home to.

I've spent every birthday with her since I was nineteen. Every year, I'd blow out the candles and make a wish. But there were no candles this time—because I didn't need them.

What more could I wish for?

I tried to tell her how much she meant to me—how she's been the perfect partner, how nothing in my life has brought me more joy, how she's made me better. But even the truest words felt small.

Unable to say it all, I let the horizon finish the sentence my heart had started.

"Look at that sky," I said. "Look at where we are—what we've done. None of this would've happened if you hadn't said yes. This past year has been the greatest of my life—and it was your gift to me."

"You helped me find myself again," I added. "This journey deepened everything good in our marriage and took our connection to a place I hadn't known was possible."

I savored that night like a final sip of rare wine—deep, unhurried, and full of meaning. I didn't want it to end. And maybe, in some quiet way, it never really will.

It was more than a birthday. It was a re-birth.

Still, endings were coming—inevitable, and near.

In nine days this trip of discovery would abruptly come to a close.

LOOP LESSONS – BIRTHDAY ON THE WATER

Crossing your wake isn't just the end of a journey—it's a reintroduction to yourself. You return different: shaped by water, refined by challenge, and softened by stillness.

The sea teaches what land cannot. Patience in the drift, courage in the squalls, grace when control slips away—these are lessons that arrive quietly, and stay forever.

You know you've grown when the small things feel sacred. A quiet passage through a lock. A glance at your partner. The sound of your own unguarded voice. Transformation isn't loud—it's revealed in peace.

Gratitude sharpens in hindsight. Looking at the one who said "yes" to the whole wild thing, you see more than a companion—you see the reason the dream was possible at all.

Some altars are made of fiberglass and quiet light. You don't need stone to mark holy ground—just a bow at sunset, where love and memory hold the silence like prayer.

The right partner turns uncertainty into beauty. This wasn't just a journey of miles, but of marriage—weathered, deepened, and re-chosen in every harbor.

Not every birthday needs candles. Some are marked by presence, not presents—by the feeling that you've lived something rare, and that the life you have is the one you'd wish for.

CHAPTER 16
THE GRATITUDE TOUR: NOTES OF THANKS

From the Tensaw anchorage we could've finished the trip in just three travel days—but we made a different choice. We decided to slow down. There was no need—and certainly no desire—to rush.

Something about this final stretch felt different. We knew it would be special.

It was pure chance—or maybe something more—that led us to buy *PATIENCE* and begin the Loop in Destin.

We could've started anywhere, but fate brought us here—to a place already rich with the sights, feelings, and memories that had first sparked the dream.

Now, as we returned, it was a chance to say thank you—to the places, the people, and the quiet influences that had shaped this journey from the very beginning.

The irony was that this stretch of coastline, so familiar by land, now felt entirely new from the water. Though we had never cruised these waters, they were deeply familiar.

The Gulf Coast had long been one of our favorite vacation spots—and now, the very place where I once dreamed of the Loop was becoming the place where our final chapter would be written.

We had driven these roads, stayed in these beach towns, made memories here for years.

But coming at it by boat—seeing it from offshore, feeling the rhythm of the waves beneath us—changed everything. The landmarks were the same, but they looked different now.

And that, I realized, was the deeper irony: it wasn't just this place that looked different. It was everything. My entire perspective had shifted.

The water had changed the way I saw the world.

Once you've lived by tides instead of clocks, measured distance in nautical miles instead of hours, and learned to trust your gut as much as your GPS, something rewires inside you.

You begin to notice wind direction, cloud movement, and the way light plays on a current. You learn to wait, to listen, to observe and react more than control.

And that alters how you see everything—land, people, even yourself.

From now on, I would always carry this watery lens with me.

Even when I returned to familiar places, I wouldn't return the same man.

The Gratitude Tour

The next nine days became a time of gratitude. A slow unfolding of thanks, honoring the people and places that had shaped our dream.

Vivid memories came rushing back—sitting at beachside restaurants, talking about "someday." I'd watch the boats drift by, aching to know what it felt like to be out there.

Now, I knew.

The next morning, on our six-hour run to Mobile, we recorded videos while the feelings were still raw and real.

We talked about how the Loop had changed us, what we loved most, what it had taught us—what we cherished, and what we wouldn't miss. (You'll find some of those posted on our Facebook group.)

As we approached Mobile, for the first time in over 3,000 miles, I tasted salt in the air.

It shimmered like a memory we could feel in our bones. I hadn't realized how much I'd missed it.

The motion changed. The wind changed. Even the birds seemed more familiar.

It felt like we were returning to the native tongue of our journey.

And then—dolphins.

They appeared suddenly, slicing through the water beside us, then dancing, leaping off the bow as if to say, *Welcome home.*

Their sleek bodies arced through the sunlight, catching golden flashes in midair before disappearing again into the blue.

Joanne laughed, her voice bright against the hum of the engine. She leaned over the bow, camera in hand, calling to them like old friends. "Look at them!" she said, beaming. "They're back!"

She filmed with one hand and waved with the other, caught somewhere between wonder and joy.

As I watched her, and I felt it too—that sense of return, of recognition, of grace.

The Gulf was welcoming us back.

Fairhope, Alabama: *A New Lens on the Familiar*

Although we'd explored much of the Gulf Coast over the years, our first stop on the return leg was Fairhope. I still can't believe we hadn't heard of it before.

This little village, founded in the late 1800s as a utopian colony, still hums with a creative, slightly offbeat energy. Artists are drawn to it, and the flower-lined streets of downtown invite you to slow down, take a deep breath, and simply enjoy the day.

How ironic.

All those years we vacationed in this region—and Fairhope was here the whole time, quietly waiting, unnoticed. How could we have missed it?

And it made me wonder: how many other things in life had been hiding in plain view?

Could this new lens—the one shaped on the Loop—help us see the familiar with fresh eyes?

Fairhope was the perfect place to offer our first "thank you"—a quiet gratitude that looked back over the entire Loop. A thank you for clearer eyes, a fuller heart, and the perspective we'd gained along the way.

It turns out, it was the perfect first stop on the Gratitude Tour.

Gulf Shores, Alabama: *Thank you, Jimmy Buffett*

On November 9, we departed Fairhope and left Mobile Bay behind, making our way to Gulf Shores.

It had been five months since we'd last seen the ICW—way back at Manasquan Inlet in New Jersey.

The water was rougher than we expected. Winds off the Gulf stirred up a frenzy, and we fought the waves as we worked our way toward the southern edge of the bay. But as we turned onto the ICW, the peninsula offered some shelter, and the waters began to settle.

We soon arrived at our next stop, Gulf Shores, Alabama—home to LuLu's.

LuLu's has locations in Gulf Shores, Destin, and Myrtle Beach—and now we could proudly say we'd docked at all three during our Loop.

LuLu's isn't just another dock-and-dine spot to me—it's owned by Lucy Buffett, Jimmy Buffett's sister, and the place radiates the same sun-soaked spirit he turned into a way of life.

Colorful, chaotic, and alive with music and laughter, it feels less like a restaurant and more like a Parrothead playground.

For us, docking at each one became a kind of unofficial milestone—a quirky little achievement on a journey built around freedom, water, and a touch of Buffett magic.

Through his music and his myth, he showed us a way to dream bigger, to live slower, to chase the horizon barefoot.

This stop was a thank-you note in person.

Jimmy Buffett's catalog was the first to awaken in me a longing for the water. His music had an easygoing sound, but underneath it was a fierce commitment to living fully.

That contrast was intoxicating.

He sang about islands and boats, sunrises over quiet harbors, and the kind of freedom most people only daydream about between meetings and mortgage payments.

Buffett didn't just tell stories—he issued invitations. He made you believe that escape wasn't just possible, it was honorable. That maybe, just maybe, you could trade in the grind for something that fed your soul.

For me, he awakened something dormant: a call to chase something bold and free. A whisper that life could be more than busy schedules and safe decisions.

That somewhere out there was a version of myself not yet discovered—waiting on the water, at the helm, salt in the air.

He sang about being alive in each moment, and he meant it.

The man squeezed every last drop out of life—and that's something worth imitating.

I was elated as we eased PATIENCE onto the fuel dock, which sits right along the ICW—fully visible to diners at LuLu's.

I'd sat in those seats before, watching other boats come and go, quietly feeling the ache of wanting to trade places.

Now, partly thanks to Jimmy, I had.

PATIENCE towered above the dock, putting us at eye level with the water-side tables. I was proud to nail the landing—smooth, steady, and right on target. It was an easy maneuver, but judging by the expressions on a few faces, it looked impressive.

As I climbed down to the dock, I could hear *"Margaritaville"* blasting on the restaurant speakers, and a chill ran down my spine.

There's no way to measure the hours I've spent with Jimmy's music in the background, shaping my dreams, setting the mood, and giving voice to feelings I didn't always know how to name.

I've been to more than twenty of his concerts over the years.

Once, in Hawaii, I crewed on a fishing boat that caught the fresh mahi for the band's pre-show buffet.

As a thank-you, they gave me a backstage pass. Unforgettable.

Another time, at a show in Vegas, Buffett gave me his wristband—just handed it to me with that signature grin.

Yeah, you could say I'm a huge fan.

But it was about far more than the music. It was the mindset. The way of life.

So thank you, Jimmy—for planting the seed, for charting the course. I might never have lived this dream without you.

Flora-Bama: *The gospel of Kenny Chesney*

Two days later, we cruised just four miles to Orange Beach. The day was perfect—beautiful water, a gentle fall sun, and Kenny Chesney singing about the *"Bar at the End of the World"* I was still riding the emotional high.

As we entered The Wharf Marina, the current picked up, and then the wind kicked in.

The harbormaster warned that docking might be tricky—but those days of white-knuckled landings were behind me.

I eased her in with quiet confidence and a grin.

After tying up, we made our way to the legendary Flora-Bama. It's more than just a bar and grill—it's become a shrine for Kenny Chesney fans.

His iconic beachfront concert, the "Flora-Bama-Jama," drew thousands here back in 2014, sealing the spot into coastal music lore.

It was a quiet Tuesday afternoon when we pushed open the door and stepped into the quirky sprawl of the Flora-Bama. The place was nearly empty—which was fine by me.

I wandered through the worn hallways, pausing to take in the many tributes to Chesney that cover the walls like sun-faded postcards from another life.

I made my way to the indoor stage—legendary in its own right—and carefully placed a PATIENCE boat sticker on the railing that frames it. Just a small mark, but a meaningful one. The crew of PATIENCE had been here.

Echoes of his music played in my head as I took it all in. Yes, I thought—I did it. I am living the life he sang about.

I'll never walk those floors again without thinking of Kenny, of PATIENCE, and of the Loop that changed everything.

Kenny's songs kept us steady during the hard miles—when the wind blew wrong, the current pushed back, and we began to question what we were doing out there.

His songs were more than a soundtrack; they were reminders of why the water called us in the first place.

Kenny sang about the soul of saltwater, and the ache you feel when you're far from it.

About unhurried days and barefoot priorities. About finding joy in stillness and peace in drift. His voice carried truths that sank deeper with every nautical mile.

What Jimmy Buffett started, Kenny Chesney finished.

Buffett gave me permission to dream. Chesney made the dream personal.

His songs—*Soul of a Sailor, Nowhere to Go, Nowhere to Be, Island Boy, Old Blue Chair,* and so many others—weren't just about boats or beaches.

They were hymns to another way of living, where the tide sets your tempo and the horizon becomes your compass.

Chesney gave voice to the feeling I now had for the water—it had become my sanctuary, my place of both adventure and peace.

Margaritaville carved the channel. *French Kissing Life* cruised it.

This is the kind of living that makes you close your eyes and whisper thank you under your breath. The kind that makes you fall in love with your own life again.

It's not a truth you can grasp from the shore. You have to feel the water lift you. Carry you. You have to go.

And now, I had.

Kenny just released a duet with Megan Moroney called, *"You Had to Be There".*

And yes, Kenny... *you had to be there.* I finally was.

LOOP LESSONS – THE GRATITUDE TOUR

Some endings deserve to be slow. The final stretch of a journey isn't always about distance—it's about reflection. Slowing down gave us time to absorb what we'd become and to say thank you along the way.

Familiar places can still surprise you. Cruising waters we had only known by land revealed how much a change in perspective can change everything. The coastline didn't change—we did.

The water leaves its mark. After living by tides and currents, you return to land with a new lens. It teaches patience, awareness, and surrender. You start to *see* differently—landscapes, people, even yourself.

Gratitude is a journey, too. Revisiting places like Fairhope, LuLu's, and Flora-Bama wasn't just nostalgic—it was reverent. Acknowledging the voices and visions that stirred this dream gave the finish line a deeper meaning.

Heroes can become guides. Jimmy Buffett lit the spark. Kenny Chesney fanned the flame. Their songs weren't just entertainment—they were invitations to a life of simplicity, soulfulness, and saltwater. We said yes.

Music matters. Sometimes the lyrics you memorize become the life you end up living. When a melody matches your soul's compass, it can carry you through storms, doubts, and long stretches of open water.

Transformation isn't just about achievement—it's about awakening. By the time we reached the end, we weren't checking a box. We were changed. And grateful.

INTERLUDE: "NOBODY DIED"

Early on, we often had an unsettling sense that we were somehow cheating death.

Inexperience. Fear. Sheer exhaustion. Most days ended with us collapsing onto the deck, grateful just to have made it.

On day seven, after a particularly harrowing stretch—split-second decisions, panicked moments, and our first stern-in docking—we pulled into Safe Harbor Pier 77 in Bradenton.

With my brother Doug along for that leg, the three of us sat numbly at the tiki hut, too stunned to speak.

After a long silence, I finally raised my glass and said, *"Nobody died."*

And just like that, we had a mantra.

From then on, "Nobody died" became our nightly toast—every evening, right to the end.

Somehow, that little phrase made its way into the broader Looper community.

Near the end—on November 1—we were anchored at the Heflin Lock anchorage, sitting on the bow near sunset, when another Looper boat came in.

They were just five days into their Loop.

We watched as they struggled to anchor—the wife on the bow doing her best, the husband at the helm loudly calling out instructions.

They finally got it set, engines off, and that's when we heard it over the VHF radio: **"That, folks, was our first solo anchoring... and NOBODY DIED."**

We laughed out loud.

It was official—we had our own phrase in the Looper lexicon.

When we crossed our wake our kids met us at the dock, waving us in. My daughters held up a sign that said, ***"You Did Not Die!"***

Nope, we actually *thrived.*

CHAPTER 17
CROSSING OUR WAKE

The Loop was complete—ten months, nearly 6,000 miles, 17 states, Canada, and a lifetime of memories packed into one floating circle.

After Orange Beach, we steered toward Pensacola—a city we'd visited many times, long before PATIENCE became part of our story.

Back then, I'd stroll the marinas, admiring the Loopers tied up for the night. I'd point, imagine, and quietly wonder if that could ever be us.

Pensacola was a seedbed.

Returning now—after living the dream—felt like opening a letter we'd once written to our future selves... and discovering it had all come true.

We stayed at Palafox Marina, nestled in the heart of Old Town Pensacola. We tied up around noon and walked to O'Riley's Irish Pub for lunch.

As we sat there, we talked about what it meant to return to Pensacola. Oddly enough, it was our first time exploring the Old Town area—and it would also be the last "new place" we visited on the Loop.

The conversation turned toward what we both knew was coming: the end. The final cruise was just one day away.

"Are you ready for tomorrow?" I asked.

"I don't think so," she said. "I'm ready to move on, but I'm not ready to finish. A lot of mixed emotions... I'm not sure how I'm going to deal with it."

We recorded that exchange, along with several others in those final days. We wanted to capture the raw emotion while it was still fresh.

I couldn't shake the weight of it. I just wasn't ready to leave this behind.

We were completely alone in Pensacola. No Loopers, no friends—nothing to dilute the moment.

The marina staff was nowhere to be found. We tied up and, the next day, cast off with no help. Just the two of us.

A year ago, that would've felt impossible. Now, it felt natural.

The Final Cruise

The next morning, we cast off for the final time. The 47-mile final cruising day looked promising. Forecasts called for light winds, with no significant chop or swell.

But forecasts aren't gospel.

As we left the marina and entered Pensacola Bay, the winds arrived—sudden and sharp. The water, so calm just minutes earlier, began to darken and lift. Small whitecaps danced across the surface, and PATIENCE rocked with the shift.

The waves hit us hard on the port beam, and soon spray was breaking over the bow.

The video from that morning catches me saying, "The last day on the Loop... and all that comes with it. Nothing good is ever easy."

That about said it all.

It seemed Neptune wasn't going to let us finish this journey without paying our final dues.

The happy news? The wind faded after a couple of hours and left us in peace.

The Golden Moment

11:42 AM, November 15, 2024.

That was the moment.

The one we'd dreamed about, talked about, quietly imagined a hundred different ways.

We knew a few family members were waiting for us in Destin Harbor, ready to cheer us in—but the real crossing, the sacred crossing, wasn't for an audience.

It was something private. Spiritual.

Nearly a year earlier, I had dropped a GPS pin—marking the exact spot where our wake began. A breadcrumb left for the soul. I wanted to be certain I would know when the circle closed.

And when we reached it, I slipped PATIENCE into neutral, letting her rest—letting her feel the stillness, the weight, the wonder of it all. This was her victory too.

I hugged her wheel and whispered thanks, praised her like the friend she was. She had carried us with grace—steady, comfortable, and sure.

Joanne and I kissed, hugged, teared up, and laughed. Our dream had become reality.

The white burgee had changed to gold.

We had changed too. We'd been shaped by storms, softened by sunsets, strengthened by challenge. Tested by wind. Refined by water. Deepened by time.

In that moment, with the wake behind us and tearful joy on our faces, we knew—we hadn't just finished the Loop. We'd become the kind of people who could.

The Loop was complete—ten months, nearly 6,000 miles, 17 states, Canada, and a lifetime of memories packed into one floating circle.

Family Celebration

After some quiet moments of private celebration, we throttled up and let PATIENCE carry us into the channel. The water turned that familiar emerald hue, and we slipped beneath the bridge one last time.

As I navigated the sharp port and starboard turns into Destin Harbor, my attention was on the busy Friday afternoon marine traffic—until a glint of movement on the docks caught my eye.

To our surprise, there they were: both of our daughters, along with Shane, Tyler, Cohen, and Charlee—smiling, waving, waiting.

Joanne was on the back deck, preparing the lines for our arrival. I tried to tell her over the headsets, but the words caught in my throat.

All I could manage was, "They're here."

They stood proudly in their PATIENCE crew shirts—the ones we gave them the previous Christmas—and Beth held up a sign that read: *"NOBODY DIED!"*

I'm so grateful my son-in-law captured the moment from the dock. I'll be able to remember that welcome forever.

We waved, we blew the horn, we laughed. We had made it.

I backed PATIENCE into the slip—right in front of Margaritaville—tied her up, and let out a long, grateful sigh.

We were home.

I don't remember tying off the lines or stepping onto the pier—I just remember arms wrapped tight around necks, happy tears, and the sound of PATIENCE resting in the slip, like she knew her work was done.

We had crossed our wake.

We changed out the burgee from White to Gold in our own little ceremony and toasted the End.

We had returned to the very place where the dream first formed, years ago. But we weren't the same people who left. We were fuller. Weathered. Wiser. And deeply, deeply grateful.

Some journeys take you far. The best ones bring you home.

But coming home doesn't make it easy to let go.

It was hard to say goodbye—to the rhythm of the water, the clarity of purpose, the simplicity of days measured in miles and marinas.

We had completed the Loop, but it had also completed something in us. And now, as the engine cooled and the boat rocked gently in her final slip, a quiet truth settled in: you can finish a journey... and still not be ready for it to end.

That evening, we celebrated with dinner in Destin, surrounded by our family. We raised our glasses, offered a few toasts, and tried to process what had just happened.

There was plenty of joy in the room—laughter, hugs, the warmth of being together—but something else lingered—quiet, unfamiliar, hard to name.

Back on the boat, as the harbor lights shimmered and PATIENCE settled into the slip, that feeling took shape.

It was sadness.

You'd think that finishing a once-in-a-lifetime journey would leave you overflowing with pride, accomplishment, maybe even relief. And it did.

But it was more than that.

It was the ache of ending something beautiful. The sorrow of leaving behind a way of life that had changed us forever.

That night, it struck me: I hadn't honestly considered what came next.

LOOP LESSONS – CROSSING OUR WAKE

Dreams worth chasing are dreams that change you. The Great Loop didn't just alter our course; it reshaped our character.

You won't be the same person at the end—and that's the point. We returned to where we began, but we came back transformed: tested, tempered, and deeply grateful.

The final miles are rarely easy—but they're almost always sacred. Neptune doesn't hand out gold burgees without asking for one last measure of respect.

Private moments mark the truest milestones. The real crossing wasn't for the crowd—it was for our souls, for the journey within.

Let your vessel be more than a tool—let her be a partner. PATIENCE didn't just carry us. She taught us, steadied us, and became part of our story.

Closure is both beautiful and bittersweet. Joy and sadness can ride the same wave—and finishing something meaningful often hurts more than you expect.

The best arrivals come with open arms and old dreams fulfilled. We were met with hugs, cheers, and laughter—but the deepest celebration was quiet, inside us.

What you return to is never quite the same—and neither are you. Home feels different after you've seen it from the sea. So do you.

You can't cross your wake without leaving something behind. And sometimes, what you leave is the version of you that never thought you could.

CHAPTER 18
AFTER THE WAKE: LIFE BEYOND THE DREAM

We had crossed our wake. The line was drawn, the circle closed. But strangely, it didn't feel complete. A part of me was still out there—adrift somewhere in the miles we'd left behind.

For so long, the Great Loop had been the dream I carried, the compass I followed. To finish it was to arrive at something I'd imagined a thousand times—like winning the Super Bowl, or summiting Everest.

And in many ways, it was exactly that.

We laughed and cheered, hugged and cried. We were proud, grateful, amazed.

But beneath the celebration, something stirred—a quiet unease I couldn't name. A feeling not of failure or regret, but of confusion.

I had finished the dream. But I hadn't truly figured out what came after it.

I went to bed that night with a gold burgee on the bow and questions in my soul—still rocking, now facing a reckoning.

The celebration in Destin lasted 3 days. Then we jumped on a plane and flew home. For the next 3 months we were back "home" in Abilene.

In the aftermath it occurred to me that much of the last 15 years had been spent in preparing, learning, fantasizing, hoping. The last year now seemed like a fog, the intensity of the trip was overwhelming at times.

But once the gold burgee was flying and the celebration faded, a new question surfaced—one I hadn't prepared for.

This turned out to be the most unforeseen part of the journey: how do you come back to dirt life without burning up on reentry?

The Weight of Reentry

The truth is, reentry after something as soul-shaping as the Loop isn't just hard—it's disorienting. The Loop wasn't just a trip. It was a different rhythm entirely. One that finally matched my spirit.

Out there on the water, time softened. Priorities rearranged. There was space to breathe, to think, to become.

And now? Now we were back on land. Back in a world where emails ding, bills pile up, and your calendar can become your boss.

I wasn't the same man who'd left. That version of me—the one who boarded PATIENCE on a chilly February morning with more questions than answers—he was gone. And the man who returned couldn't just plug back into the old life.

Because the plugs didn't fit anymore.

That's the part no one warns you about: how the adventure changes you. How it strips away the unnecessary. How it wakes up desires that don't correlate with the old self.

The Loop forces you to confront your weaknesses. It exposes your edges. And it gives you a choice: change, or fight it the whole way around.

I made a conscious choice—to not resist the change, but to embrace it.

So, when we got back to Abilene, Texas, I felt unmoored again, but this time in a different way.

Not from the water. From the land.

A Different Kind of Tired

You don't just get tired from the journey. You get tired from what it reveals. The Loop stretched us. It tested our systems, our relationship, our faith, and our sanity. But it also simplified everything.

No lawn to mow. No TV shouting the news. No rush-hour traffic or HOA meetings. Just currents, clouds, charts, and the occasional engine alarm to keep you humble.

I enjoyed that freedom. I thrived in that simplicity. So now, when I walk back into the commitments I once accepted as normal, I feel resistance. Not because I'm lazy. But because I know the price. I know what it costs to carry obligations that don't align with your values.

The Loop showed me how much life I was missing under the weight of maintenance, meetings, and mindless routines.

The good news? I now get to choose—carefully and intentionally—what lines I tie to the dock. Some commitments, I'll never make again.

The ones I keep now are the ones that truly matter. They're chosen, not inherited or assumed. I don't ever want my life to be that overcommitted—or that frantic—again.

These days, my pace is more deliberate. My priorities are clearer. And my world orbits the things that give it meaning: family, faith, and joy.

Joanne's return home was different.

Throughout the Loop, I rarely thought about what came next.

She often dreamed of land—of home—of the life waiting beyond the water. She imagined a place where she could land gently—something fresh, something grounded. For her, the dream of the Loop was always intertwined with what came after.

For me, the Loop *was* the dream.

Dirt Life

The Looper term for the world beyond the water is "*dirt life*". It's almost vulgar to me. It sounds harsh, jarring, mechanical. Because after the Loop, land feels like that. Heavy. Loud. Angular.

You don't realize how much the water has softened you until you try to slot yourself back into the old life—and everything feels too sharp, too fast, too much.

Dirt life keeps calling you back, like a habit you thought you'd kicked. But you've seen what it feels like to be free. You've tasted a new rhythm. And even if you go back, you'll never see it the same way again.

I think that's the true impact of catching a dream: it doesn't end with the dream. It ends with *you,* transformed.

The Mirror

On the Loop, I met myself. That sounds overly poetic, maybe even dramatic, but it's true. The Loop was a mirror. It showed me what I value, what I fear, and what I want more of.

It forced me to admit the areas where I was still trying to prove something—to others, to myself, maybe even to God. It peeled me back to the bone.

And it gave me space to build again—on something more honest.

The water taught me patience. The weather taught me humility. The people taught me generosity. And solitude taught me how to listen again—both to God and to my own heart.

So when I sat at that dinner table in Destin, with a half-eaten steak and a gold burgee firmly in my grasp, I wasn't just celebrating the end of a journey. I was mourning the end of a season. One I can't return to in the same way.

Because even if we Loop again—and we might—it won't be the same. *I won't be the same*. You only get one first Loop.

The Collision of Selves

Maybe the hardest part of coming home is the collision between your old self and your new self. The man who left had dreams, doubts, blind spots, and a sense of control that was largely imagined.

The man who returned had been refined. Humbled. He'd seen fog close in and friendships open up. He'd felt the quiet power of nature and the loud cracking of strain and stress.

You can't unknow what you've learned.

That collision—between who you were and who you've become—is where grief takes root.

Now the rhythm I'd once trusted—the one that rocked me gently into who I became—was silent. But it still lived in me.

You can't unfeel the stillness, unsee the sunsets, unlearn the lessons. And trying to live like you used to is like shoving a new soul into an old suit. It doesn't fit.

Heaven on Earth

Sometimes I think the Loop was a glimpse of heaven. No, it wasn't perfect. We had bad weather, engine problems, and days when we snapped at each other.

But the rhythm of the water matched my spirit in a way that nothing on land ever had.

I imagine that's what heaven will be like—perfect harmony, unhurried and whole.

If you were in that kind of place, at peace, and someone asked if you wanted to return to earth, wouldn't you just smile and say, "Why would I ever leave?"

I think that's why finishing the Loop felt so heavy. Because it was like waking up from a beautiful dream—and wondering if the real world will ever feel quite right again.

Plugging In

One of the unexpected gifts of the Loop was the clean slate it gave us when we returned home. As I've mentioned, leaving meant unplugging from our former life—routines, obligations, even some relationships.

That kind of purging wasn't easy. But the Loop gave us a legitimate reason to step away from almost everything, and in doing so, it created a rare and powerful opportunity: when we came back, we could be intentional about what we plugged back in.

I've been especially inspired by books like *The More of Less* by Joshua Becker, who wrote,

"The first step in crafting the life you want is to get rid of everything you don't."

Now that we're easing back into land life, I can feel the calendar filling up fast. But this time, I'm being more selective. I'm choosing commitments that reflect what I truly value—things I *want* to give my time and energy to, not just things I feel obligated to do.

Anne Lamott put it perfectly:

"Almost everything will work again if you unplug it for a few minutes... including you."

The Loop was just that—a full-system reset. Stepping away gave me the space to breathe, reflect, and rethink what I actually want my life to look like moving forward.

The result?

More peace. More purpose.

I wake up with a sense of direction, not dread. Yes, my schedule may someday be just as full as before the Great Purge—but now, it's filled with things that nourish me, stretch me, and bring joy.

Things that matter.

So here's a simple but powerful challenge: Make a list of all the things you're doing that you *wish* you didn't have to. Then ask yourself: *What would happen if I just... didn't?*

What if you gave yourself permission to unplug—and only reconnect to what actually fuels you?

Maybe you're thinking, "That sounds nice, but I can't walk away from all of it." And I get that.

Our year away made it easier—"out of sight, out of mind" is a real thing. But even if you can't disappear for a year, you can still press pause. You can still choose to suffer the initial guilt that comes with letting go—and then experience the freedom that follows.

Life After the Loop

So what do you do when you catch your dream?

You remember. You write. You tell the story. And you live differently because of it.

You don't try to go back to who you were. That version of you is done.

You honor him—thank him for being bold enough to chase the dream in the first place. Then you ask the new version of yourself what he wants to do with all that he's learned.

For me, that's writing this book.

It's also how I show up with my family. How I think about work. How I make space for silence. How I say yes—or no—with more clarity and less apology.

I still have days where I ache for the water. Where I'd trade everything for one more sunset at anchor, one more coffee at the helm, one more VHF call from a buddy boat.

But I don't resent the ache.

It reminds me that something real happened.

That I was fully alive out there.

And that I can be fully alive here, too—if I carry the rhythm with me.

The Final Lesson

The Loop was never just about boating. It was about becoming.

You don't have to do the Loop to experience this kind of change. But you do have to chase something honest. Something big enough to scare you and clear enough to guide you.

You must be willing to leave the dock—not just literally, but emotionally and spiritually.

You must let go of what's comfortable so you can find what's true.

When you do, you just might catch your dream.

And if you're lucky—it will catch you, too.

I passed through the five stages of grief when I returned to land. Only recently am I reaching the final one: acceptance.

Now, I'm ready to tuck the Loop into a sacred place in my heart—always cherished, always accessible.

Whenever I'm tempted to drift back into old patterns, I'll close my eyes and remember those precious days on America's Great Loop.

LOOP LESSONS: AFTER YOU CATCH THE DREAM

Finishing the Loop may feel more like loss than triumph—and that's okay. Grief and gratitude can coexist at the end of something beautiful.

Reentry takes grace. Be patient with yourself—and with those who didn't take the journey with you. They won't fully understand what changed, and that's not their fault.

You won't fit back into your old life exactly as you left it. The Loop reshapes you. Let the new shape stand.

Freedom comes with a cost—and a calling. The kind you tasted out there may challenge what you're willing to recommit to on land.

Your dream changes you only if you let it. Don't rush back to what was. Reflect, recalibrate, and move forward with intention.

Honor who you were—but give space for who you've become. Integration, not imitation, is the goal.

Crossing your wake is not the end. It's the beginning of living with bold heart, blue mind—and deeper purpose.

CHAPTER 19
BUILDING A BETTER BOAT

The Song That Found Me

Last night, I sat alone in the hot tub beneath a wide West Texas sky. Steam curled into the air, blurring the edges of the moon.

A light breeze rustled the mesquites, and somewhere in the distance, a coyote called—soft and familiar.

The scent of the ranch drifted across the fields, still warm from the day's sun.

I wasn't expecting anything profound—just a quiet soak to end the evening, music playing low in the background.

And then, as if on cue, Kenny Chesney's *Better Boat* began to play. I'd heard it a hundred times before. But this time, it felt different.

This time, he was singing about me.

The lyrics spoke of being alone but not necessarily lonely, of learning to be still, of letting time do its healing work.

Line by line, it felt like Chesney wasn't just singing a song—he was naming the ache I hadn't yet been able to voice.

Not grief, exactly.

Not regret.

Just that deep, unshakable feeling you get when the best chapter of your life has ended... and you're not quite sure what comes next.

The more I listened, the more I saw how the song gave shape to everything I was feeling but hadn't yet articulated.

So, I started paying attention to the themes—because they weren't just lyrics. They were lessons.

Solitude vs. Loneliness

In the seven months since we crossed our wake, I've spent a lot of time alone—reflecting.

The solitude has been valuable, giving me space to absorb the impact of the journey. But it's not a place I want to live long term.

There's a difference between choosing time alone and living with loneliness.

These days, loneliness seems woven into modern life. We're endlessly connected by technology—yet rarely face to face.

After a year of dockside conversations, shared sunsets, and spontaneous chats on the water, the contrast is jarring.

Back on land, it feels like we've forgotten how to truly connect. We pass each other in silence, heads down, distracted.

It's no wonder so many people feel like something's missing—because something is.

The Grief of Returning

Chesney's lyrics go on to describe how recent months have brought changes that don't always feel easy yet bring growth. That hit home.

The last few months have brought more change than I expected.

West Texas is a long way—mentally and emotionally—from the Loop. And I've come to realize just how much your environment shapes how you live, how you think, and how you feel.

Adjusting hasn't been easy. It takes time to accept what coming back really means.

I'll be honest—when we first returned, it was almost unbearable. The loss hit harder than I imagined.

The Loop wasn't just a journey; it had become a way of being. And leaving that behind left a quiet emptiness I can't seem to shake.

Sometimes, I catch myself forcing a smile when someone asks, "Aren't you glad to be back home?" But in my heart, I'm thinking, *this isn't home.*

And in that moment, I feel deeply disconnected—from them, and from the life I'm supposed to resume.

It still hurts.

Grief catches me off guard—a scent, a photo, a random text from a Looper friend—and the pain rushes back in. When that happens, all I can do is breathe and try to smile.

Breathing and Remembering

But it is slowly getting better. I must let time do its work.

One line in the chorus centers on the simple rhythm of breathing in and out—and I've clung to that.

When I miss the lifestyle—which is often—I slip into the hot tub or hop on my bike. It's the same bike that carried me over 600 miles during the Loop, and now it's one of the few ways I can still feel the wind, the movement, the rhythm of that life.

I breathe and remember. Exhaling as I recall the peace, the joy.

The Loop will always be a place in my mind where I can retreat. As I age, I can only imagine how wonderful it will be to have this special place in my memory.

I will lose many freedoms and abilities, should God grant me many more years of life, but nobody can take this away from me.

I did it. I completed the Loop. I lived it. Nothing can change that now.

Conversations That Still Matter

The song also reflects on having friends who let you talk through what's still broken. I know that feeling well.

I still have many Loop friends I stay in touch with—people I can call to talk about the journey. Friends who *get it* because they lived it too. Turns out, they suffer the same wounds.

We talk about the things that still don't work:

How hard it is to return to dirt life.

How we're struggling to squeeze back into the old shoes of home.

How the new man is wrestling with the old one.

How even the people we love grow tired of hearing us talk about it.

We talk about what's still hurting:

How much we miss the water, the people, the sense of discovery.

How impossible it feels to move past the grief.

How we wish we could stop comparing—but can't.

It's hard to get excited about lunch at the same restaurant for the thousandth time or biking the same loop you've ridden a hundred times before.

The thrill is gone—and with it, the discovery.

And yeah—that stings.

The Isolation of Unshared Experience

When I visit with my old friends, I understand why they don't want to hear it. They just can't relate.

It even hurts to know that PATIENCE is sitting somewhere in a marina, without me. She was home.

I understand now what Chesney meant when he sang that boats are a vessel of freedom.

Now, the pain of losing that freedom is real. My Looper friends know it, and so do I.

There are so many things I still wrestle with. The traffic. The dry, dusty wind. The absence of water nearby.

I live 400 miles from the coast—but it might as well be a million. Some days, it feels like I'm a lifetime away from the life I really want.

I catch myself looking at people as they busily shuffle through dirt life and I wonder if they ever dream of more.

I wish I could grab them and shake them and explain what they may be missing.

"How can this be enough," I want to scream to them.

A Love You Don't Want to Lose

Maybe that's the feeling you have when you lose a loved one. After the funeral, people forget. They see you and they don't mention the loss anymore.

That's how it feels to have lost the Loop. It almost makes me angry at times.

I don't want to forget. I don't want to move on.

I want to remember.

Chesney sings about learning to let go, at least a little—and I'm starting to.

Sometimes—just for a moment—I let go of the hurt and the loss... and I manage a real laugh.

After the Dream Comes the Question

And then I think of those old Super Bowl interviews, when the confetti is still falling and the athlete is asked, "You just won the Super Bowl—what are you going to do now?"

The answer: "I'm going to Disneyland!"

I used to smile at that. But lately, I understand it on a deeper level.

What do you do after you've achieved your dream? One you planned for, prayed for, poured your heart into?

What could possibly be more?

I'm trying to find a place to keep the Loop—inside me—where I can honor it, carry it, even be shaped by it... without letting it weigh me down.

Riding the Waves You Can't Control

Another line in the song speaks of learning to ride the waves we can't control.

I'm starting to understand that some things from the Loop can't be recreated. They can't be replaced. They can only be remembered—and honored.

And I'm slowly making peace with that.

The Loop taught me to accept what I can't control. And the truth is, much of what I'm struggling with now—this return to land life, this sense of disconnection—can't be fixed by force.

One quiet day at a time, I'm trying to live the lessons the water gave me.

If the Loop taught me anything, it's that control is mostly an illusion.

Weather, current, tide, breakdowns—you can't stop them. You can only respond with grace, patience, and presence.

Life is no different.

The world I've come back to is the canvas I've been given. I can't repaint it to look like my year on the water—but I can still add new color, new texture, and shape a life that reflects what I've learned.

One that still carries the heart of the Loop.

I may no longer wake with the bow facing a pink-lit horizon, but I still chase that kind of light, wherever I am.

The Better Boat

The song ends with a line about building a better boat. And I think that's the heart of it.

It's taking time.

I hate the waiting. Waiting for what's next, waiting for life to recalibrate.

Waiting for the mourning to end. But it will.

I don't hold PATIENCE's wheel anymore. In fact, she's not even called PATIENCE now.

Like me, she's moved on.

"PATIENCE," I keep telling myself. Just remember, PATIENCE.

And I do, every day.

You might think I'm complaining. But I'm not.

It's hard to change—especially when I spent decades living with a Red Mind: always alert, always on, always pushing forward.

It took a full year of immersion—of salt air, quiet mornings, dockside friendships, and anchorages under stars—to begin softening that part of me.

To begin shifting from Red Mind to Blue.

And now, back on land, I'm learning how to carry that change with me.

Truthfully, it's not easy to let the Blue Mind lead in a world driven by noise and speed.

But I want to.

I want that peace to become part of me—not just something I experienced on the water, but something I carry wherever I go.

Not just a chapter in my story. A new way of being.

So yes—I am growing stronger than I was.

I'm learning to let God work in this moment—this strange, unsettled space between who I was before the Loop and who I'm becoming now.

I'm trusting Him to take everything I experienced out there—the joy, the storms, the solitude, the friendships—and distill it into something lasting.

Something deeper.

I believe He's shaping me into a better man—not because I earned it or figured it all out, but because I was willing to be changed.

I said yes to the water. Now I'm learning to say yes to the waiting—trusting that what's being built in me will be stronger in the right places, and lighter in the ways that matter.

The Loop didn't just alter how I see the world—it altered how I'll move through it.

As I navigate whatever comes next, I know my boat—my life, my spirit, my mindset—will be more seaworthy than before.

More balanced. More resilient. More aligned with what truly matters.

And in a world so full of storms, with tides that shift without warning, I'm going to need every bit of that strength.

The seas ahead may not be calm. But I'm not the same man who left the dock. And now... I'm building a better boat.

LOOP LESSONS – BUILDING A BETTER BOAT

Solitude can heal, but connection sustains. The quiet after the journey gave space to reflect—but human connection is still essential. We're not meant to live in isolation.

Returning is harder than setting out. Re-entry into "normal life" after the Loop can feel like grief. The true challenge is learning how to carry the transformation forward.

Not everyone will understand—and that's okay. The people who didn't take the journey can't fully relate. But that doesn't diminish its worth.

Memories are anchors, not weights. Holding onto the beauty of the Loop isn't about clinging—it's about honoring what shaped you.

The old self doesn't fit anymore. After profound change, trying to wear your former life can feel like walking in shoes that are too small.

Even after the dream ends, the journey continues. Life after the Loop still has meaning—especially if you keep building something with what you learned.

Control is an illusion. Response is everything. Just like on the water, life's storms can't always be avoided—but they can be navigated with presence, grace, and patience.

Transformation takes time—and trust. Growth doesn't happen on a schedule. Letting God do His quiet work in the waiting is part of the voyage.

You can't relive the Loop—but you can live differently because of it. The goal isn't to recreate the trip. It's to let it reshape how you live every day.

Your best vessel is still being built. With the Loop behind you, life ahead may still be uncertain. But your boat—your soul, your mindset—is stronger, wiser, and better than before.

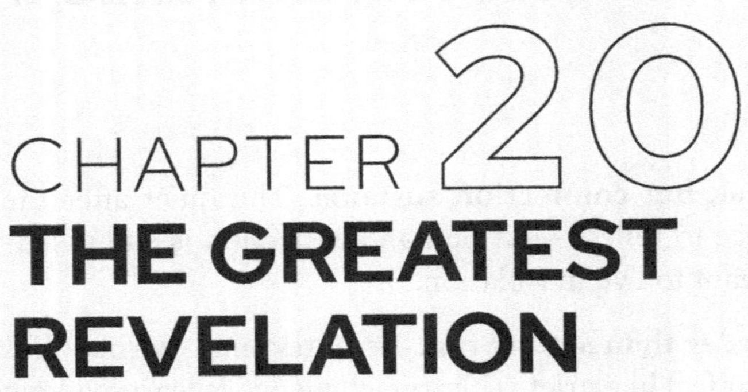

CHAPTER 20 THE GREATEST REVELATION

Not Just Alive—Living

I didn't understand it at the beginning—maybe I couldn't.

We set out chasing a dream: a 6,000-mile adventure, a chance to live one of mine. But I soon discovered something unexpected. The real treasure of the Loop wasn't in completing it.

It was more complex than that. More divine.

Remember the revelation I couldn't hand you in the Prologue?

At first, I thought the big truth was simple: *It's not in the achievement—it's in the pursuit.* And that's close. But I confused the thrill of the chase with something even deeper. I was circling the truth, but not quite landing on it.

As the miles passed, it began to come into focus.

I wasn't just racking up experiences. I wasn't just living more adventurously or interacting more deeply with the world.

A new man was being formed in me.

Bear with me while I try to put it into words—though I admit, I still wrestle to capture it.

Live While You're Alive

Jimmy Buffett sang about people who live lies and ultimately regret it. I know that feeling all too well.

Because here's the truth: when you dare to chase your dreams, you open a door. And on the other side, you meet a version of *you* that only exists if you say yes to the pursuit.

If you don't take that chance—not only do you settle for a lesser life—you live with regret. And regret is a quiet, steady rot.

We talk a lot about addiction—alcohol, drugs, screens—but the greatest addiction I see is complacency. It numbs. It softens your edge. It whispers, *"This is fine. It's not great, but it's not terrible. Just stay here. Don't risk it. Don't hope too big."*

That lie is lethal. It kills slowly and silently.

We all know the line: *"To thine own self be true."* I would add this: *"Be true to your heart—or you'll never become the 'self' you were put here to be."*

You don't need a life that looks good on paper. You need one that feels true in your bones.

The Sacred Act of Pursuing

Don't worry about failure—not as the world defines it. Settling is the real failure. Not falling short. Not making a mess. Not even quitting halfway. The greatest loss is never having tried.

Because there is something sacred about the pursuit—something electric in the act of moving toward your dream.

You don't have to summit Everest or sail the world. You just have to do the most you can with what you've been given, right now.

And that's enough.

The goal isn't the finish line. It's not the flag or the fanfare. The real prize is what happens *through* the pursuit.

The trying. The reaching. The decision to leave the couch and go do the thing.

That's where the joy lives. That's where your spirit stretches. That's where regret dies—and meaning is born.

It's Not Too Late

It's not too late. It's not too small. And it's not too far gone.

There's a Loop waiting for you—whatever it looks like. Start where you are. Give what you can. Move forward, even if it's just one quiet mile at a time.

Because the greatest tragedy isn't failing.

It's never beginning.

God-Given Dreams

Maybe your dream is simple: grow a garden. Write a story. Start painting again. Find your voice. Whatever it is, God put it there. It's part of your design.

If you let it starve from neglect, you won't just lose a hobby—you'll lose a piece of yourself.

You don't want to be on your deathbed asking, *"What if?"*

Because here's what I've come to believe: The dreams we carry inside us aren't random. They're not frivolous, shallow, or foolish.

They're sacred.

They are signals—divine echoes of who we were made to become. Not every desire. Not every passing impulse. But the *deep dreams*—the ones that keep whispering through the noise of life—*those* matter.

They're not distractions from your purpose. They *are* your purpose, waiting to be awakened.

They aren't there to entertain you. They're there to *form you.*

The Greatest Revelation

Because in the pursuit of those dreams—not just the achievement, but the courageous pursuit—something essential unfolds.

You become more patient. More alive. More awake. You stretch in ways you didn't think possible. You deepen. You transform.

That dream isn't just about what you might accomplish.

It's about who you must *become* in order to reach for it.

And if you ignore it—if you bury it beneath busyness, fear, or the comfort of *"maybe someday"*—you don't just miss an opportunity. You miss a version of yourself that never fully gets born.

Because if you never chase what calls you...you'll never meet the real *you*— the one God intended to be created through His design, and your effort.

LOOP LESSONS – THE GREATEST REVELATION

The finish line isn't the reward. The true prize is who you become on the way.

God-given dreams aren't random—they're roadmaps to your transformation.

Pursuit is sacred. Forward motion awakens something holy inside you.

Regret is born not from failure, but from never beginning.

Settling is its own kind of death. Comfort can be the enemy of becoming.

You were designed for more than safety. There's a version of you that only emerges through risk.

Small dreams matter. Write the story. Plant the garden. Find your voice.

Dreams are not for entertainment. They are divine tools of formation.

It's not too late. It's not too far gone. Begin with what you have.

If you never chase what calls you, you'll never meet the real you—the one God intended through His design, and your courage.

EPILOGUE: THE WAKE WE LEAVE BEHIND

We crossed our wake—and with it, a threshold. The Loop ended, but something deeper had only just begun.

We had been told the journey would change us. I know that now. Not just because of the miles, the locks, or the technical skills we sharpened—but because somewhere along the way, the water got into my soul.

It smoothed out the sharp edges. It softened what had grown hard. It reminded me that control is an illusion, time is a gift, and presence is the only real currency.

This was so much more than I expected. It was a full-body baptism—into stillness, into motion, into the sacred intersection of dreams and daily life.

We learned to read the sky. To listen to each other. To forgive more quickly and laugh more often.

I discovered new truths about myself, and rediscovered old truths I'd nearly forgotten.

And we did it together.

When people ask what I'll remember most, it's not the stats or the stops. It's the feeling.

The early morning light on calm water. The sorrow of saying goodbye to good friends. The sound of my wife's laughter echoing across the bow.

The quiet awe that came over me when I realized: we're really doing this.

We didn't just circle a continent. We peeled back the layers of ourselves. And in doing so, we uncovered what matters most.

Gratitude isn't strong enough a word. Reverence might be closer.

Because this journey—this gift—reshaped everything. How I view time. How I define success. How I love, rest, listen, and dream.

We returned to the dock changed. Saltier, yes—but also more whole.

And though we've stepped back onto land, the Loop hasn't let go of us. I don't think it ever will.

February 12—that was the day we packed up all our belongings and walked off *PATIENCE* for the last time.

I lingered, not wanting to let go. I walked out onto the bow late in the day and sat for just a moment.

The sun was beginning to set, and the water granted me a beautiful farewell.

The gold burgee was still fluttering gently in the breeze. *PATIENCE* swayed ever so slightly—like a mother rocking a child. Comforting me.

I carefully removed the gold flag, handling it like a fine garment.

I whispered a prayer of gratitude. *PATIENCE* had been the perfect boat for us.

She carried us safely for 6,000 miles.

Like a mother sheltering a child, she seemed to know what we didn't. She knew the way—somehow avoiding the disasters that lurked in the water—and always seemed to know the right places to stop.

I felt like a son leaving home—nurtured, prepared, and quietly carrying the weight of all he'd been given. Confident, but marked forever by the hands that shaped him.

There was one last thing I had to do.

I took one final look inside, brushing my hand along every surface, trying to let go.

Then I opened a cabinet—one tucked out of sight—and with a marker, I scribbled a simple thank-you note:

"*PATIENCE*, **thanks for the joy you brought me.**"

I signed and dated it. And I hope it stays there until the end.

Call it melodramatic to personify a boat—but I don't care.

She was more than fiberglass and engines. She held memories of past Loops. And now, she holds ours.

If you're wondering whether it's worth chasing your own version of this dream—my answer is yes. Absolutely yes.

But know this: it will ask more of you than you expect... and give back more than you can possibly imagine.

Crossing your wake isn't the end. It's not a finish line—it's reentry.

Into a changed life, with a changed heart, and a new way of moving through the world—with hands that still remember the helm.

FINAL REFLECTIONS – LOOP LESSONS FOR LIFE

The Loop wasn't just a route on the water—it became a compass for living. These are the deeper truths I'll carry with me, long after the miles are behind me:

Start before you're ready. Growth doesn't wait for perfect conditions. The journey begins the moment you say yes—ready or not.

Fear fades with motion. Most of what we feared dissolved the moment we moved. Action shrinks anxiety faster than overthinking ever could.

Progress often hides in the messy middle. Some days felt slow or unclear—but they still moved us forward. Not all transformation feels like momentum.

Your partner is your most important crew member. The Loop tested our marriage and strengthened it. Grace, honest words, and shared laughter mattered more than perfect docking.

Stillness reveals what motion conceals. Slowing down uncovered what really matters. Some of our greatest discoveries surfaced in the quiet.

Nature has a voice—if you're willing to listen. Water, wind, and wildlife became our guides. We learned to read the sky, interpret the current, and find meaning in silence.

Community is a lifeline. Fellow Loopers reminded us that no one does this alone. Advice, encouragement, and companionship made the journey richer.

Control is an illusion. The weather, the current, the breakdowns—we couldn't control any of it. Peace came when we surrendered and adjusted, not when we resisted.

Beauty is everywhere when you're present. A sunrise at anchor, a dolphin off the bow, a quiet hand on the helm—these were the rewards that mattered most.

Crossing your wake isn't the end. It's not a finish line—it's reentry. Into a changed life, with a changed heart, and a new way of moving through the world.

GLOSSARY OF NAUTICAL & LOOP TERMS

AGLCA *America's Great Loop Cruisers' Association, an organization supporting boaters doing the Great Loop.*

Anchor *A heavy object dropped from a boat to the bottom of a body of water to keep the vessel from drifting.*

Anchorage *A designated or suitable spot to drop anchor and remain stationary, often protected from wind and current.*

Beam *The widest part of a boat, typically measured at the middle.*

Burgee *A flag flown on the bow of a boat*

Bow *The front section of a boat.*

Cleat *A metal or plastic fitting on a boat or dock used to secure ropes (called lines).*

Docktails *A social tradition among Loopers involving cocktails and conversation on the dock, usually at day's end.*

Fender *A cushion-like device hung between a boat and a dock (or another boat) to prevent damage during docking.*

Flotilla *A group of boats traveling together.*

Galley *The kitchen area on a boat.*

Great Loop *A roughly 6,000-mile boating route that circumnavigates the eastern United States and parts of Canada via rivers, canals, and coastal waterways.*

Helm *The steering station of a boat, where the wheel or controls are located.*

ICW (Intracoastal Waterway) *A protected network of channels and bays running along the Atlantic and Gulf coasts of the U.S.*

Line *A rope used on a boat for docking, anchoring, or securing items.*

Lock *A section of a canal with gates at both ends that raises or lowers boats between stretches of different water levels.*

Looper *Someone who is actively cruising or has completed America's Great Loop.*

Marina *A dock or basin with moorings and facilities for yachts and small boats.*

Mayday *A distress call used over marine radio to signal a life-threatening emergency, such as sinking or fire.*

PATIENCE *The name of our boat—our home during the Great Loop journey.*

Port *The left-hand side of a boat when facing forward.*

Slip *A parking space for a boat at a marina, typically between two docks or pilings.*

Starboard *The right-hand side of a boat when facing forward.*

Stern *The rear part of a boat.*

Trawler *A type of motorboat designed for long-distance cruising, often with a displacement hull and fuel efficiency.*

VHF *Very High Frequency radio, used by boats to communicate with marinas, bridges, locks, and other vessels.*

Wake *The waves created behind a boat as it moves through the water.*

CREDITS

Front Cover Photo
Joanne Tackett

Back Cover Photo
Mark Rohlffs

Jacket Design
James Graham

Medical and Health Support
Dr. Kevin Finley

Mechanical and Technical Support
Mike Hogeland

Family
From my parents to my daughters and grandchildren, each of you gave something up to make this journey possible. Thank you for releasing us without guilt, for carrying us through the hard times, and for sharing the joy in countless calls and visits. This book—and this adventure—could not have happened without you.

ABOUT THE AUTHOR

Mike Tackett is a lifelong entrepreneur, storyteller, and adventurer. He has spent decades building companies in real estate, renewable energy, and retail electricity. His career has taken him from diving for freshwater shells in the Tennessee River to developing utility-scale wind and solar projects in Texas.

In 2024, Mike and his wife Joanne set out aboard their 39-foot yacht *Patience* to complete America's Great Loop, a 6,000-mile waterway journey through the heart of the United States and Canada. The voyage reshaped his understanding of time, identity, marriage, and the joy of chasing dreams. *Blue Mind, Bold Heart* is his first book, blending memoir, reflection, and adventure.

Mike and Joanne live in Abilene, Texas, where they continue to share stories, music, and a love of water.

APPENDIX A

OUR LOOP ITENERARY

(FLORIDA)
2/3/24- Destin, 2 Georges
2/6/24- Panama City, Emerald Harbor
2/7/24.- Apalachicola, Scipio Creek
2/8/24- Dog Island. ANCHORED
2/9/24- Tarpon Springs, Mar Marina
2/10/24- Clearwater Municipal Marina
2/14/24- St. Pete area ANCHORED
2/15/24- Bradenton, Safe Harbor #77
2/16/24- PATIENCE was on the hard at Snead Island Boat Works
2/29/24- Blackburn Point Casey Key Marina
3/2/24- Cabbage Key, ANCHORED
3/3/24- Marco Island, ANCHORED
3/4/24- Key West, Galleon
3/8/24- Long Key, ANCHORED
3/9/24- Miami, Venetian Yacht Club
3/11/24- Hollywood Beach, ANCHORED
3/12/24- Pompano Beach, Pier #32 Lighthouse Marina
3/13/24- Jupiter Florida, Anchored at Tiger Woods -ANCHOR
3/14/24- Fort Pierce, City Marina
3/20/24- Mosquito Lagoon, ANCHORED
3/21/24- Palm Coast Marina
3/23/24- St Augustine, River's Edge Marina
4/1/24- Sisters Creek, Free Dock

(GEORGIA)
4/2/24- Jekyll Island Jekyll Island Marina
4/7/24- Sunbury Crab Company
4/8/24- SavanahIsle of Hope Marina

(SOUTH CAROLINA)
4/13/24- Hilton HeadHilton Head Harbor Marina
4/15/24- Beaufort, SC Safe Harbor, Beaufort, SC
4/17/24- Charleston Courtyard Marina
4/19/24- Charleston Safe Harbor (moved marinas in Charleston)
4/23/24- Georgetown, SC Hazzard Marina
4/24/24- Myrtle Beach, SC Barefoot Marina
4/25/24- South Port, Deep Point Marina
4/26/24- Swansboro, Church Street Town Marina

(NORTH CAROLINA)
4/27/24- Beaufort, NC Town Creek Marina
4/30/24- Oriental Oriental Marina and Inn
5/2/24- Belhaven Marina
5/3/24- Alligator River Marina
5/4/24- Coinjock Marina

(VIRGINIA)
5/5/24- Porstmouth, VA, Tidewater Marina
5/8/24- Yorktown , Riverside Landing
5/10/24- Deltaville, Ragatta point Marina
5/11/24- Reedville, Crazy Crab Restaurant
5/12/24- Solomons Island Yacht Club

(MARYLAND)
5/17/24- Tighlman, Knapps Narrows Marina
5/18/24- St Michaels Marina
5/22/24- Kent Island Yacht Club
5/29/24- Annapolis, Capital Yacht Club
6/1/24- Rock Hall Landing Marina
6/3/24- Havre De Grace, Tidewater Marina

(DELAWARE)
6/6/24- Delaware City Marina
6/7/24- Cape May, New Jersey, Utch's Marina

(NEW JERSEY)
6/10/24- Atlantic City, NJ, Golden Nugget
6/11/24- Manasquan, Bills Landing
6/12/24- Hudson Point Marina

(NEW YORK)
6/16/24- Cortlandt, Cortlandt Yacht Club
6/17/24- Kingston Hudson River Yacht Club
6/18/24- Erie Canal, New Baltimore Shady Harbor
6/19/24- Erie Canal, Albany Yacht Club
6/30/24- Erie Canal, Schenectady, Donavan's Mohawk Harbor
7/1/24- Erie Canal, St Johnsonville Municipal Marina
7/2/24- Erie Canal, Rome NY, Rome City Free Dock
7/3/24- Erie Canal, Brewerton, NY, Winter Harbor Marina
7/18/24- Erie Canal, Oswego Marina

(CANADA)
7/19/24- Rideau Canal, Kingston Mills Lock Wall
7/20/24- Rideau Canal, Lower Brewers Lock 45
7/21/24- Rideau Canal, Jones Falls
7/22/24- Rideau Canal, Chaffeys Lock Wall
7/23/24- Rideau Canal, Upper Brewers Lock Wall
7/24/24- Rideau Canal, Kingston Mills Lock Wall
7/25/24- Kingston, ONT, Confederation Marina
7/26/24- Trenton, Trent Port Marina
7/29/24- Trent Severn Waterway, Frankford
7/30/24- Trent Severn Waterway, Trent Hills, Old Mill Park
7/31/24- Trent Severn Waterway, Hastings Lock 18
8/1/24- Trent Severn Waterway, Peterborough, City Marina
8/4/24- Trent Severn Waterway, Lakefield Lock 26
8/5/24- Trent Severn Waterway, Buckhorn, Lock 31
8/6/24- Trent Severn Waterway, Bobcaygeon, Lock 32
8/8/24- Trent Severn Waterway, Rosedale - Lock 35

8/9/24- Trent Severn Waterway, Thorah - Lock 40
8/10/24- Trent Severn Waterway, Port Orillia
8/12/24- Trent Severn Waterway, Big Chute - Lock 44
8/13/24- Georgian Bay Midland, Bay Port Yacht Center
8/14/24- Georgian Bay Frying Pan Bay, Canadian Park
8/15/24- Georgian Bay Henry's Fish Restaurant, Sans Suici
8/16/24- Georgian Bay Parry Sound, Big Sound Marina
8/21/24- Georgian Bay Wright's Marina, Britt, ONT
8/22/24- North Channel, Sportsman's Inn
8/24/24- North Channel, Little Current
8/25/24- North Channel, Benjamin Islands -ANCHOR
8/26/24- North Channel, Blind River Marina

(MICHIGAN)
8/27/24- Drummond Island Yacht Haven
9/3/24- Mackinac Island State Harbor
9/5/24- Charlevoix City Marina
9/10/24- Leland Township Harbor
9/12/24- Jacobson Marina Resort
9/13/24- Ludington Municipal Marina
9/14/24- Muskogen, Safe Harbor Great Lakes
9/15/24- Safe Harbor Tower Marina, Saugatuk

(INDIANA)
9/17/24- West Basin Marina, St. Joseph

(ILLINOIS)
9/18/24- Washington Park Muni, Michigan City
9/20/24- DuSable Harbor, Chicago
9/24/24- Joliet Free Wall
9/25/24- Heritage Harbor, Ottawa
9/30/24- East Port Marina , Peoria
10/1/24- Beardstown, Tug dock
10/2/24- Hardin, dock at Mel's
10/3/24- Grafton Harbor
10/6/24- Alton Marina
10/7/24- Kaskaskia Lock

10/8/24- Diversion Channel - ANCHORED
10/9/24- Angelo Towhead - ANCHORED

(KENTUCKY)
10/10/24- Paducah City Dock
10/11/24- Green Turtle
10/18/24- Panther Creek- ANCHORED

(TENNESSEE)
10/19/24- Paris Landing State Park Marina
10/20/24- Pebble Isle Marina
10/22/24- Clifton Marina

(MISSISSIPPI)
10/23/24- Grand Harbor

(ALABAMA)
10/26/24- Florence Harbor Marina
10/28/24- Aqua Yachts, Iuka
10/29/24- Midway Marina
10/30/24- Columbus Marina
11/1/24- Heflin Lock Oxbow Anchorage ANCHORED
11/2/24- Demopolis, Kingfisher Marina
11/4/24- Bashi Creek Anchorage
11/5/24- Bobby's Fish Camp
11/6/24- Tensa Anchorage ANCHORED
11/7/24- Fairhope Marina
11/9/24- Homeport Marina, Lulu's
11/11/24- The Wharf Marina, Orange Beach

(FLORIDA)
11/14/24- Pensacola, Palafox Marina
11/15/24- Destin, Harbor Walk Marina
11/17/24- Destin (Shalimar) Two Georges

Made in the USA
Coppell, TX
17 January 2026